LINGUA EX MACHINA

Books by DEREK BICKERTON

Lingua ex Machina
Language and Human Behavior
Language and Species
Roots of Language

Books by WILLIAM H. CALVIN

Lingua ex Machina
The Cerebral Code
How Brains Think
Conversations with Neil's Brain*
How the Shaman Stole the Moon
The Ascent of Mind
The Cerebral Symphony
The River That Flows Uphill
The Throwing Madonna
Inside the Brain*

*with GEORGE A. OJEMANN

Lingua ex Machina

Reconciling Darwin and Chomsky with the Human Brain

WILLIAM H. CALVIN
DEREK BICKERTON

A Bradford Book
The MIT Press
Cambridge, Massachusetts
London, England

First MIT Press paperback edition, 2001
Copyright ©2000 by William H. Calvin and Derek Bickerton

WilliamCalvin@alum.mit.edu
http://faculty.washington.edu/wcalvin

Derek.Bickerton@worldnet.att.net

Supplements and corrections can be found on the web page
http://WilliamCalvin.com/LEM

This book was designed, and set in Palatino, by William H. Calvin; it was printed and bound in the USA.

Library of Congress Cataloging-in-Publication Data

Calvin, William H., 1939-
    Lingua ex Machina: Reconciling Darwin and Chomsky with the human brain / William H. Calvin, Derek Bickerton.
        p.   cm.
    "A Bradford book."
    Includes bibliographical references and index.
    ISBN 0-262-03273-2 (hc. : alk. paper), 0-262-53198-4 (pb)
    1. Neurolinguistics. 2. Brain–Evolution. 3. Chomsky, Noam. 4. Darwin, Charles, 1809-1882. I. Bickerton, Derek. II. Title.
QP399.C35   2000
612.8'2–dc21   99-33464
                                                                              CIP

Contents

Linguistics is arguably the most hotly contested property in the academic realm. It is soaked with the blood of poets, theologians, philosophers, philologists, psychologists, biologists, and neurologists, along with whatever blood can be got out of grammarians.

–RUSS RYMER in The New Yorker, 1992

That the ultimate answer in a long-lasting controversy combines elements of the two opposing camps is typical in biology. Opponents are like the proverbial blind men touching different parts of an elephant. They have part of the truth, but they make erroneous extrapolations from these partial truths. The final answer is achieved by eliminating the errors and combining the valid portions of the various opposing theories.

–ERNST MAYR, This is Biology, 1997

1

The Villa Serbelloni
Bellagio, Italy

Derek,

People at dinner last night kept asking me what Chomsky's innate grammar is all about. Where is this language macromutation in the brain, and all that?

Wrong question, of course, but it's a sure sign they've gotten used to the amazing view of Lake Como from the terrace where we eat at the Villa Serbelloni, on a long table with several dozen interesting people. You'll see when you arrive. If there's a clear evening before I get back from Milan, remember to watch for the last of the sunset over the Dolomites.

Provided, of course, the other "residents" give you a chance. Several confessed to reading up on our subject, in anticipation of our arrival for a month of writing about the brain and language. It forcefully reminded me that Chomsky's innateness has been the intellectual spectator sport of the last four decades. I tried to explain to them that some gene-specified aspect was unsurprising to a biologist – that you and I hoped to flesh it out with appropriate anthropology and neuroscience in a way that

Chomsky wasn't particularly interested in doing, and to provide some evolutionary proposals that wouldn't rely on macro-mutations and the like.

I also tried to explain your notion of protolanguage put forth in *Language and Species*, with a good supply of words but with sentence length limited to only a few words by the lack of structural elements such as phrases and clauses. Protolanguage has no way of saying who did what to whom, not without an enormous effort. I emphasized that there was a large gulf between protolanguage and our full-fledged syntax without any obvious intermediate states, quite a jump from my pidgin Italian to being able to nest four verbs in saying, "I think I saw him leave to go home."

It's going to be challenging for us to try and describe how the gulf was first bridged by evolutionary processes. I hope we can avoid the *deus ex machina* quality of some of the previous attempts to explain the origins of language ability, the ones that finally seize upon a slender, unsupported reed as *the* way out of the muddied morass – the equivalent of that "god machine" the ancient Greek playwrights wheeled in to solve thorny plot problems. Yet it is a language machine we're searching for, one capable of those elaborate maneuvers seen in language with syntax (you don't have to think about it; indeed, you can't turn language recognition off), but conforming to some design constraints imposed by the neurobiology (what it's possible to do with mere neural circuits) and the evolutionary history (up from apelike communication and mental powers in only five million years, each stage bootstrapping the next).

But, in a broader view, language is just our best example of the whole range of higher intellectual functions. Our *lingua ex machina* probably needs to be able to handle creative shaping up of quality (for instance, figuring out what to do with the leftovers in the refrigerator), long-range planning, procedural games, and even music. Solve the structural basis for one, and you might solve them all.

I think that the linguists' conceit, that syntax is what thought is all about (and that without syntax, you couldn't think with any depth or originality), reflects a useful strategy for brain researchers, simply because syntax provides a lot of useful constraints on theorizing. But other parts of higher intellectual function might be even more useful in that regard. Want to lay any bets that we would discover more about higher intellectual function via studying music in the brain? Yes, music seems likely to be a spare-time use of the neural machinery evolved for thought and language – but we might be able to separate the issues of vocabulary and structuring better in music, where you have structure without predication, as the Israeli musicologist Ruth Katz reminded me at dinner! What's unmusical in any culture might tell us what the neurons can't do.

Intelligence (in our sense of versatility in dealing with novel situations) is a particularly intriguing part of the puzzle of higher intellectual functions. But as Ernst Mayr once said, most species are not intelligent, which suggests "that high intelligence is not at all favored by natural selection" – or that it's very hard to achieve. So our look at bootstrapping syntax also needs to keep in mind this more general problem of finding indirect ways of achieving intelligence. What gives rise to syntax might also give intelligence a big boost.

Evolution, after all, is full of sidesteps, such as those conversions of function that Darwin identified. Wheelchair considerations may be what "paid for" all of those curb cuts on every corner, but most of their subsequent use involves wheeled suitcases, baby carriages, grocery carts, skateboards, bicycles, and other uses that would never have paid for it. Some of the underpinnings of language may be secondary uses as well, so we need to watch for free "curb cuts" affecting syntax.

See you soon.

Bill,

Well, when I got greeted with a facetious "Calvin tells us that the two of you are going to out-Chomsky Chomsky," I started to wonder what you'd been telling them. Then I remembered that whatever you tell people about Chomsky, they seem to get hold of the wrong end of the stick. Some people get no respect, others get no comprehension. If what Chomsky said about innate capacities had been said about any species but ours, everyone would have accepted it years ago. The evidence that language is a biologically determined, species-specific, genetically transmitted capacity is simply overwhelming, no matter how many people try to chip away at isolated bits of it. But somehow humans are supposed to be special. The same rules don't apply. The idea that our prize possession, language, is just some mechanical thing seems very threatening to some people.

Unfortunately, Chomsky is unwilling to look either at the neurological infrastructure of language or at the ways it might have evolved. *Why* he's unwilling is neither here nor there. That's his business. No one has to do everything. But obviously, once it's established that language is biologically determined, the next step is for someone to try and find out exactly how it evolved. And once it's established that language is rooted in the structure of the brain, the next step is to go looking for it there. These three things – language, evolution, and the brain – it seems to me, are interlocking. You can't really look at any one of them without looking at the others. If you want to know how language evolved or how it operates via brain mechanisms, you've got to know exactly what it's *like* – how it differs from bee dances and chimp calls. But you really can't be sure what it's like until you've seen how it evolved or how it works in the brain. All three areas of knowledge should be feeding one another, but they're not. And that's the king-size hole in our understanding of ourselves that I'm hoping, between us, we might be able to plug up a bit in the next month.

However, once we start looking at how language could have evolved and how the brain does the job, we become aware that some of the ways linguists have looked at language are more than a little awkward. Over the last decade or so, an enormous amount has been written about the evolution of language – all the more enormous when you consider how little we know about it. Some of what has been written is sensible; much, alas, is not. To go through this literature, to evaluate it, to show how our ideas differ from it, would be an enormous task, one that would inevitably get in the way of the concrete proposals we have to make. So we're not going to go through it and we're not going to criticize anyone else's approach. In the endnotes we'll show where alternative answers can be found.

Derek,

Well, Chomsky's term "language organ" might have been unfortunate, as was some of the early supercharger-type imagery used to describe how language might have been tacked onto an ape brain, as were the cardboard notions of how evolution works (those *deus ex machina* macromutations). But I have no quarrel with what I take to be the heart of Chomsky's argument, that human brains are predisposed to use certain types of syntax and not other possible schemes – and that it wasn't obvious how to do this from textbook versions of Darwinism. Today, we'd probably emphasize a baby's predisposition to *discover* patterns in the language (or *invent*, in the case of creoles) and thereby softwire a language machine in one of the neurologically possible self-organizing schemes, rather than speaking of something being innate from conception onward. But that's just the current state of the ever present nature-nurture debate.

There are lots of little brain areas, the size of a small coin, one of whose functions is particularly specialized – say, naming inanimate objects. I'll give some examples when I eventually discuss where concepts are located in the temporal lobe. We still tend, following Gall's phrenology, to give functional names as if an area were exclusively concerned with the named function. But most areas are multifunctional; we merely discover one function that compels our attention – and name the area after it! And so onwards to the reification fallacy (it has a name, therefore it must be a thing).

But certainly the language specializations of the brain are not exclusive; the same areas of brain have a lot to do with inventing oral-facial and hand-arm movement sequences, and with judging sound sequences – and these functions probably all evolved together. Their brain real estate may well constitute a common facility, one used not just for language tasks but for any involved sequence, whether sensation or movement or thought – just as curb cuts are now multiple-use though paid for by a single use.

Structure is one way to look for the physical basis of real language, but you can also ask how each individual develops the functionality during early life. Part of the language instinct could turn out to be something very simple – say, a real fascination on the part of the young human with discovering any hidden patterns in the sensory environment, such as the repeated strings of speech sounds that we call words. We may happen upon crystal-like self-organizing tendencies in the neural circuitry that preserve them – tendencies that aren't likely to come from experience. That way, after discovering words in the auditory barrage, you can go on to discover the pattern of words that we call a "question." There could be one stage after another of searching for higher- and higher-order patterns, each making use of the same automata propensities in the neural circuitry.

So language acquisition might consist of the discovery of patterns in the environment, some of which can be remembered by patterns in the brain. Just as some types of crystal are more common than others, so syntax might settle into certain patterns more than others. Those patterns are what, I take it, "Universal Grammar" refers to. Rather than a gene for a language machine, you might have an epigenetic tendency to seek hidden patterns in your sensory environment which, together with the brain's potential for creating varied "crystals" shaped up by previous evolution, would give you the syntax that makes us so different from the apes.

NOW, DEREK, LET ME SUMMARIZE what we said about book organization at breakfast and afterwards, when we walked up to the castle on the cleaver. I need a little *aide memoir* for my fallible brain, the sort of thing that politicians write in their diaries to save for the day when they write their memoirs.

We're not trying to write *the* book about language origins, one that covers the landscape of interesting ideas that float around at conferences on language origins. We'll be happy just to show several powerful ways of getting from ape behaviors to syntax without relying on the usefulness of communication per se. We're after invention, not improvement.

Our imagined audience is not unlike the other residents here at the Villa Serbelloni: the typical serious reader, but not necessarily in the sciences (the artists and poets hereabouts ought to find it of interest and be able to follow our explanations). As for content, well, as Ernst Mayr likes to say, the big scientific questions tend to resolve around *what*, *how*, and *why*. And they're all interlocking; one's incomplete without the others (though we often pretend otherwise, as when we focus on one aspect at a time as "the answer"). So we might want to structure our Bellagio book around the relevant what-how-why questions.

What's a word, anyway? What's a simple utterance of a few words? And, since a longer sentence is not just a heap of words any more than a house is merely a heap of construction materials, what's all this argument structure and phrase structure that constitutes syntax – or used to, back before minimalism struck? And what about all those little closed-class words of grammar, such as the articles and prepositions? What are the stages of a child's development of language?

How does the brain represent a word? How does it link words up? How does it store new memories, retrieve them? How does the brain invent a novel utterance, without it being complete nonsense most of the time? How does language deteriorate in strokes?

But all the linguistic *what*'s and neurophysiological *how*'s are incomplete without the evolutionary *why*'s, those step-by-step explanations about how things came to be the way they work now, explanations involving Darwin's bootstrap. Why is it unlikely that words evolved out of primate cries and calls? Why did our particular kind of syntax evolve? Does it have anything to do with the brain expanding fourfold during the ice ages?

What's our best scenario for a step from primate cries to protolanguage? From lots of vocabulary up to the use of syntax for facilitating long sentences like this one? We'll need to talk about the relationship between evolving language and all the other changes evolution made in the typical ape (I know you want to discuss the extensive advance in sharing food and doing favors for friends). Then, with some examples in hand, we ought to discuss what would constitute a really satisfying explanation, covering the whole spectrum of such questions about language and the rest of the higher intellectual functions that separate us from the smartest apes. The "unfinished agenda," as it were.

THOUGH OFTEN CONSIDERED as a gradual series of improvements in efficiency, evolution is also characterized by a string of Good Tricks conserved by evolution and reused in different contexts. Many biological structures are multipurpose, and the most obvious "function" of a structure may change over time. Darwin's example was the swim bladder of the fish, most obviously useful for adjusting buoyancy via filling up a balloon with blood gases, but also useful as an interface for exchanging blood gases with the atmosphere, a simple lung that might allow the fish to crawl ashore. Darwin may not have known about curb cuts, but he spoke of a conversion of function, and warned that selection favoring one function might well benefit another function. We'd probably say that selection for language abilities benefitted musical abilities, because it's so hard to figure out what evolutionary circumstances would have rewarded four-part harmony. There may be no free lunches in some ultimate sense, but there sure is a lot of bundling of products; pay for one, get something else "free." And the minor product may turn into the major one in the long run, enormously aided by the initial natural selection that paid – in a different coin – for the other.

Also, because structures are so easily duplicated, once you have the genes for one, it is possible to specialize in several directions at once. Our chromosomes are filled with non-functional near-duplicates of the functional genes; that's exactly how any computer programmer would operate, doing experiments on copies of the functioning program, eventually using the new one more and more of the time as the bugs are eliminated.

Simple rules generate complex patterns. (The big lesson of fractals and chaos!) Some variants on the existing rules are stable (most are nonsense, others quickly undo themselves), and so one sees self-organizing systems bootstrapping themselves in what Jacob Bronowski calls stratified stability. The stabilities are, of course, somewhat confining – just as the steep fjordlike walls of the Como valley made it easier for the ancient glacier to go certain directions rather than in others.

That's the sort of thing we ought to see with language evolution: experimental advances above a plateau of stable function (like your protolanguage), sometimes discovering a new stable level (like structured utterances), but with confines developing as you go.

LEVELS OF ORGANIZATION are, fortunately for us, a commonplace in technology. As an example of four levels, *fleece* is organized into *yarn*, which is woven into *cloth*, which can be arranged into *clothing*. Each of these levels of organization is transiently stable, with ratchetlike mechanisms that prevent backsliding: fabrics are woven to prevent their disorganization into so much yarn; yarn is spun to keep it from backsliding into fleece.

A proper level is also characterized by "causal decoupling" from adjacent levels. For example, you can weave without understanding how to spin yarn (or make clothing). Many of the branches of science are founded around a single level of organization. Mendeleyev figured out the table of elements and predicted the weight and binding properties of undiscovered elements, long before anyone knew about atomic spectra or biochemistry. As a chemist, it helps to know the electron orbits that underlie chemical bonds, and it may help to understand an overlying level such as stereochemistry, but most of chemistry is a set of relationships within a level – just like weaving, a subject in its own right.

Within the brain sciences, we have to cope with close to a dozen levels of organization (and so we frequently argue about whether learning is a matter of gene expression, ion channel, synaptic, neuron, or circuit-level alterations). We can even invent new levels on the fly, such as analogies, though most of them don't last for very long.

But some do. Among the major tasks of early childhood are the discovery of four levels of organization in the apparent chaos of the surrounding environment. Infants discover *phonemes* and create standard categories for them. With a set of basic speech sounds, babies start discovering patterns amid strings of phonemes, averaging nine new *words* every day. Between 18 and 36 months of age, they start to discover patterns of words called phrases and clauses, adding *-s* for plural, adding *-ed* for past tense. After *syntax*, they then go on to discover Aristotle's rule about *narratives* having a beginning, middle, and end. Thus in four years, children "pyramid" four levels of organization, each with its own rules that are causally decoupled from the underlying level's rules. I'd caution that levels don't mean orderly hierarchies: you might have several different levels taking off from an earlier one, more like a tree or a web than a ladder.

It is tempting to treat consciousness as the highest level of organization that you've currently got cooking. When you first contemplate the toothpaste in the morning, the level of consciousness might not be very high, operating merely at the level of objects or simple actions. Handling relations (such as speaking in sentences) may become possible only after your morning coffee. The relations between relationships level (analogies) may require a double espresso. Poets, of course, have to compare metaphors, which requires a series of stage-setting preliminaries. Writers attempt to dramatically shape their materials to result in, as Sven Birkerts said in *The Gutenberg Elegies*, "a kindled-up sort of high."

Understanding such staging might allow us to spend more time at more abstract levels – or even invent a new level in this house of cards, if the prior levels can be sufficiently shored up. I can almost imagine a meta-poet taking a long walk here at the Villa Serbelloni, trying to stage manage yet another level atop the earlier shaky edifice, inventing meta-metaphors.

So, Derek, I wonder if your protolanguage isn't just going to be a level of relationships – mostly associations between a few objects and a verb – atop which syntax can operate as a new, more structured level. And that some sort of meta-syntax could operate atop it, in turn.

WHAT YOU WANT THE NEURO to provide, as I understand it, is a nice clear step up from protolanguage to syntax, the brain finally getting its act together because of one important improvement that, together with what's already in place, provides an emergent property, syntax. The committee can finally do something that all the separate parts couldn't. It might be like adding a capstone to an arch, which permits the other stones to support themselves without scaffolding – as a committee, they can defy gravity. Our task as scientists is, in part, to imagine the scaffolding that could have put such a stable structure in place initially.

I can imagine some Good Tricks that might provide that big step, allowing for the recursive nature of embedded phrases and a considerable improvement in speed of operation. A big step doesn't necessarily mean that performance suddenly flowers. Graded improvement of function can still occur via the amount of time that you utilize the Good Trick, or the number of situations to which you apply it, or the intensification of culture occasioned by widespread use (more vocabulary invented, etc.). But I think that I can give you something without intermediate syntax levels, something that will deteriorate back to protolanguage in a fairly obvious manner without intermediate stops (I've never heard of an aphasic patient able to embed two deep, but not three). And that recursive phrases and clauses will emerge in our *lingua ex machina* as neatly as they do in the child's third year.

DB: I know that you like to make fun (as do I) of attempts to leap from the sub-basement of quantum mechanics to the penthouse of consciousness, but doesn't biological psychiatry attempt to leap from a gene to a psychosis?

WHC: Ah, the "gene" for schizophrenia. But such things merely show that a high level is dependent on the whole edifice. A crack can indeed propagate upwards through a dozen levels. Just as sparkplug failure causes an occasional traffic jam, so a misread gene can occasionally set up a psychosis. But if you want to understand the typical traffic jam in the middle of nowhere, you have to understand how the packing density of vehicles moving at somewhat different speeds can, in combination with a hill to climb, create a traffic jam even where there is no traffic entering or leaving the freeway. So, too, understanding delusions and hallucinations means knowing how thought builds on the immediately-underlying layers of the edifice. We'll need to "stand under" thought and appreciate how network dynamics are structured by syntaxlike processes, so we can nest sentences. That a bad gene can disrupt it simply doesn't explain very much. Useful explanations require *relevant* foundations, not just another "everything is connected to everything" demonstration.

2

What Are Words?

Bill,

Okay, I'll start off with what's a *word* – and with why primate utterances aren't really words, because they can't be combined with others for a new meaning.

Were someone asked what a sentence was, the reply would almost certainly include something about words – that a sentence consisted of words strung together, or something of that sort. But when you think of words, what are they exactly? The word "word" seems to have some sort of intermediate existence between, on the one hand, very concrete terms like "table" and "chair" and, on the other, very abstract ones like "chore" and "nothing."

On the one hand, "word" differs from "table" and "chair" in that we can say, "This chair is made of wood, that one of metal, that table of plastic," and so on. We can't say the same about any of the various referents to which "word" may be applied. Any word may appear in a variety of guises: as sound-waves between a mouth and an ear; as marks on a page; and – in some sense yet to be defined – as things we have in our brains. We can remember words, forget them, confuse them with one another – in short, perform on them any of the operations we can perform on any of the things in our memory store.

On the other hand, we are able to say that words consist of something. They're not like chores; anything can be a chore, depending on how you look at it. They're not like nothing, which can't be like anything. And there's a still more dramatic difference between 'word' and any other word. The word "chair" is not a chair, and the word "chore" is not a chore, but the word "word" is a word. So what on earth can we mean when we talk about words? Of course, everybody knows what a word is, but again, it's like knowing what a sentence is. We know one when we see one, but when it comes to saying what it actually is, the problems begin.

For, of course, the whole evolutionary purpose of gathering, storing and filing such impressions is to be able to identify things. If we identify an orange as an orange, we then know that we can eat it without harm. If we identified an orange as a deadly nightshade berry, we wouldn't eat it, and would be deprived of its nutritive value. If we identified a deadly nightshade berry as an orange, we might eat it, and might die as a consequence. So it's very clear that the correct identification of things in the world – correct in terms of the consequences we predict from them, rather than in any sense of absolute truth – is adaptive, in the evolutionary sense of the term.

That is, if you identify things correctly, you survive and (hopefully) reproduce, breeding descendants able to identify at least as well. If you don't identify correctly, you are slightly more likely to die before you reach reproductive age, and your misidentifying genes will not make it as far into the future. However slight an edge you get from correct identification, it's all you need to ensure that in a few hundreds or thousands of generations, most members of your species will identify things at least as well as you did, while most who were worse at it will be long gone.

Of course, the example I gave is absurdly simple; most creatures can distinguish between things that resemble one another far more than do oranges and deadly nightshade berries. And because of their evolutionary value, these processes of identification, these fine discriminations in terms of stored sensory impressions, began very early in evolution, long before mammals walked the earth, or dinosaurs, indeed long before the first sea-creature, balancing perilously on its fins, dared to trespass on a still barren and desolate dry land. In us, those processes may seem to have reached a higher pitch of refinement (though organisms as diverse as bats, pit-vipers, and electric eels have highly developed senses that we do not possess even in rudimentary form). But they are in no way different in type from the processes that operate in other species, including species we might fancifully suppose to be considerably "lower" than we are.

So LET'S TRY A SLIGHTLY DIFFERENT APPROACH. Let me state the minimal conditions that a neurological model of how words are represented has to meet in order to be plausible, in light of what we currently know about language. Those conditions will be, so far as I can make them, neutral with respect to whatever theory of language one may hold – Chomskian, functionalist, whatever. (There are a few things that linguists can agree on, though you might not think so if you heard them arguing.)

A word is, as one might expect after all this, something multifaceted. In order for a word to function, it has to trigger off a concept in the hearer's mind. If the speaker says "orange," this has to activate some kind of concept of orange in the hearer's mind. Otherwise it would be as if I said "naranja" and you didn't know Spanish.

Two problems here. The first is general, but I want to sidestep it, for the moment, at least: that is, *what a word actually represents*. A naïve view is that it represents an object – "orange" represents an orange, or oranges. But then what do words like "absence" or "nothing" represent? Ferdinand de Saussure said, no, words represent concepts. But since we still can't be sure what a concept is, that doesn't help too much. For the moment, let's just say that words represent something, somehow. They serve to focus your mind on some aspect of reality – or rather, I should say, of the picture of reality you carry about with you in your brain.

The second problem is more specific to the example given, though it affects a surprising number of words in any language. Take the two sentences, "She ate an orange" and "She wore an orange sweatshirt." It should be clear now why "orange" can't just mean an orange – it can mean a color.

(Yet an orange doesn't have to be orange to be an orange – unripe oranges are green.) In other words, when you hear the string of sounds that make up the word "orange," you can't tell simply from these if it's the fruit or the color that the speaker intended to evoke. You have to determine what role the word plays in the sentence, whether it stands alone as a noun or modifies some other noun, like "sweatshirt."

Another way of putting this would be to say that words have *properties*. Properties are things like, what word-class does a given word belong to (adjective, noun, verb, and so forth), whether it has to have a complement and if so what kind (for instance, prepositions must have a noun-phrase as complement), whether it has any agreement features ("she" for instance is singular, third-person, and feminine, as well as nominative case) that have to match up with others in the utterance, and so on. The brain's representation of a word has to include all of these things somehow, as well as more obvious things like meaning. To date I don't think we have much idea about precisely how this is done. It looks as if where a word is stored in the brain might be determined by word properties, but for most features we don't even have that much of a clue. However, it's clear the brain must represent words somehow, or we couldn't talk. It's reasonable to suppose that both "oranges" have separate representations even if the sound-pattern that they share is the same.

So let's consider for a moment just "orange" as a noun. When you hear the word "orange," this may suggest to you just some vague picture ("kind of fruit") or it may evoke the taste of an orange, or its color (ripe or unripe), or its smell, or the texture of its skin, or – if you happen to be a fruit-grower here in Italy – probably also the soft thud that an overripe orange makes when it falls and hits the ground, as well as probably lots of other things that might seem obvious to Italian fruit-growers but lie wholly outside the knowledge of you and me.

NOW LET'S GET RID OF A PSEUDO-PROBLEM that worries lots of people. How can words work if they evoke different things in different people? How can people ever understand one another? Well, in most cases at least, however little a word evokes in my mind, that little will be a subset, however weird or limited, of the set of things that the same word evokes in the minds of those who are expert in the relevant field. If it isn't – if the word "orange" evoked in me some of the properties of bananas – we're in real trouble. But this seldom happens, and if it does, we conclude there's something wrong in the brain of the person concerned.

Back then to "orange" and the things it may evoke. What these things are are basically sensory impressions – but not of one particular object on one particular occasion. Rather they are generalized impressions derived from various occasions of seeing oranges, tasting them, and so on. If such impressions were not accurately filed in the brain somehow, we might see an orange on one occasion, note and observe it, see another, note and observe that, and fail to realize that they belonged to the same category.

Each of these sensory impressions will be linked to a particular sense. However, if one receives a combination of sense impressions with any degree of frequency, or with less frequency but in a life-threatening manner (the sound of a charging lion's roar, for example, coupled with the sight of the animal getting rapidly larger), it's hard to see how any member of the combination could subsequently occur without potentially triggering the others. In other words, in addition to representations in terms of a single sense, you get representations in terms of several sensory modalities – cross-modal representations.

The importance of this, for our purposes, is that not so long ago some believed that the reason animals didn't have language was that they didn't have cross-modal representations. Obviously, if you have words you have to have cross-modal representations. The word "lion" wouldn't be of much use to you if it evoked only the smell of a lion and not its appearance, or only its appearance and not the sound it made. Not that it has to evoke all of these at once – simply that it has to be able to, if needed, if you are going to get all the mileage out of words that you would like to get.

WHC: No problem with multimodality representations, Derek. Many of the neurons of association cortex, and some of the ones in the primary sensory cortices, respond to several major modalities of sensory input. For example, neurons in somatosensory cortex may also respond to light. But there's some point in emphasizing the difficulty of multimodality linkups, because of the problem of doing them on-the-fly, when dealing with some combination that you've never encountered before (and so couldn't have established any specialist connections for the combination). Language tasks are full of novel combinations.

While there aren't objects in the brain, like those in the compartments of the left-luggage office, there are ensembles of neurons that effectively represent objects, analogies, and the other bricolage of our mental life. Yes, a person is only a collection of molecules, but their pattern of organization is everything; it's the well-functioning organization which is the difference between a living person and a cadaver. My mental representation of "apple" is only a collection of neurons, all of which are also used for other purposes on occasion. Still, they form an organization that functions pretty well for recognizing apples, eating apples, pronouncing "apple," and so forth.

It's hard to talk about representations in the brain, how we memorize something and later make use of it, because of the lack of ready analogies in the technological world. Our memory isn't much like that of a computer memory (though it does have some functional equivalents of keyboard buffers, short-term RAM, and long-term hard drives). Ours doesn't have any empty slots because it's a distributed, overlapped type of storage where the new stuff has to fit in, amidst the redundant resonances for a lot of old stuff. To appreciate how memory works requires talking about nearly a dozen different levels of organization (most areas of science only have to deal with several). All those levels – molecules and their receptors and channels, membranes, synapses, neurons, minicolumns, macrocolumns, areas, and larger brain regions – exhibit self-organization and emergent properties; they are all involved in any explanation.

For now, suffice it to say that concepts with fuzzy edges are what you'd expect from the sensory neurophysiology. This will not make lawyers happy, nor others that like to dissect issues into smaller and smaller well-delineated fragments, but nature seems to like fuzzy edges, at least at the cellular level of organization. Precision is accomplished with large committees redundantly trying to do the same task; precision is often an emergent property of enough imprecise neurons. I suspect that there's a strong link between the neural process that makes syntax possible and that which makes our speculative, beyond-the-animals consciousness possible – namely, that they are both founded on the Darwinian cloning competitions of cerebral cortex. More later.

Some people use "thought" to mean "mental image," but most mental images are pretty abstract, what makes cartoon sketches so successful. I'd use "thought" in a broader sense, allowing relationships such as analogies. Relationships are far more abstract than objects themselves, and there are often layer upon layer of abstractions in our metaphors, undoubtedly aided by syntax's structuring. Thoughts also follow themes, such as searching for cause and effect: I often approach various problems with what, overall, might be considered a Darwinian template, looking for signs of a spread of variants, some of which survive and reproduce better than others.

Note that to represent a word, a cross-modal representation must also have at least two other characteristics. It must not be an association that is automatically triggered whenever what it refers to appears – or rather, if is triggered, it must be possible to inhibit it from triggering its spoken representation, otherwise every time we saw a dog we would be obliged to say "dog." And the association must not trigger an automatic response, or be limited to a single kind of response. Whenever someone says, "Pass the salt," we don't want to have to choose merely between passing the salt and not doing anything. We might want to throw the salt at them, if it was the last in a long chain of similar requests, or we might want to say, "Get it yourself," or make any other of a potentially infinite number of responses. In other words, coming or going, words have to be decoupled from the world of action in ways that animal calls are not. For instance, vervet monkeys can, on sighting a martial eagle, either give the martial eagle warning or keep quiet, but if the warning is given, the vervets seem to have no other choice than to do nothing or to run up a tree. Maybe they could do other things, but the evidence makes it look as if the action of running up a tree is preferentially linked to that kind of warning. Words cannot not have this property if they are to work as words should. True, a word in a particular context might be so linked – if someone shouts "Fire!" in a crowded theater, we are more likely than anything to head for the door – but if we ran out of the room every time the word "fire" occurred in casual conversation, we would be regarded as weird indeed.

The representation of a word has to be hooked up with things other than preferential responses. It has to link with all the different sensory representations of whatever it refers to. It has to link with memory in such a way that any relevant remembered item can trigger it. It has to be linked, potentially, with representations of other words, so that longer utterances can be formed. It has to be linked preferentially with whatever sounds give it a phonetic realization. But it mustn't be linked with particular responses, or indeed any responses. Words may seem on occasion to precipitate action, but in fact are only part of the evidence on which choices of action are made. If someone tells us to go, we may or may not go; if we do, a whole set of other considerations will have conspired to drive us. That's certainly one of the most crucial differences between words and animal calls.

WHC: Most of the animal calls are analogous to our exclamations; they're usually emotion-laden utterances. Chimps in the wild have about three dozen characteristic vocalizations, all in this category; some easily translate into "Whoopee!" or "Weird!" or "Get away." They have some signals, such as maintaining eye contact (between gorillas, this is a threat; between bonobos, a sexual invitation). Carrying a stick or waving leaves may be used to invite playful romps. There are many expressive body postures and movements, some of which carry directional information, as when a chimpanzee drags a branch down a path that he wants others to follow ("Let's go this way!") or swings it behind the stragglers to herd them.

Some vocalizations may be repeated to intensify the meaning, but otherwise combinations of calls and cries have no additional meaning, in the manner of combinations of our elementary vocalizations, the phonemes. Indeed, one of the evolutionary puzzles is how our ancestors made the transition from a few dozen vocalizations, each with an assigned meaning, to our present system of meaningless phonemes (about forty in English), that have meaning only in combination with each other. Even novel combinations (never seen before words like "bumbleberrism") can be easily handled on the first pass.

One-word (or one-stock-phrase) utterances are often the only things that aphasics can speak after their left lateral language areas have been damaged in a stroke. Total mutism usually requires damage to the supplemental motor area, just above the corpus callosum in the brain's midline, an area implicated in monkey vocalizations. So we may want to think of standard exclamations – and most primate calls – as involving an older, more primitive system, located far away from those left lateral brain areas that seem to be important in our kind of syntactic language.

The primitive exclamation speech area may not even be the cortical system where the first words (meaningful units that are recombineable for additional meaning) were invented; cortical areas near the Sylvian fissure seem more likely to have housed the first words. It makes you think in terms of a second language system, operating in parallel with an older one, and not necessarily an intensification of the first system. The second system could have its origins in something like face recognition and social relationships, rather than producing vocalizations.

Right. The amazing thing is that some people still believe that language must have developed out of some kind of hominid call system. In that case it would be strange indeed that the hominid call system – screams, crying, laughter, finger-pointing, fist-shaking and the like – still continues to exist alongside language.

Moreover – since this section concentrates on the unit *word* to the exclusion of all larger units – we're not saying much here about a still more sharply distinguishing feature of words. What would be the use of a language that was limited to single-word utterances? Words must be potentially able to combine with one another, at least in the minimal subject-predicate mode: you use the first word to focus the hearer's attention on a class or class-member and the second to make some kind of comment on that class or class member (dogs bark, John left . . .). You can't do this with calls, because each simply triggers readiness for a certain behavior, and each requires a different behavior. There's no way two calls can ever be linked with one another in the way that words can, so that the second call would say something about the first.

But a question we maybe should ask at this stage is whether the representations of words are simply cross-modal sites, places where the different sensory impressions can come together – something like what I think Damasio means by "convergence zones" – or whether they require more abstract representations as well. The more abstract representation would serve as a further buffer between sensory input and motor output. I think in order to answer this we would probably need to know more about how both human and other primate brains work. Other primates can have cross-modal associations, but an association isn't a representation, per se. Maybe you can't get from cross-modal association to cross-modal representation without having a word or sign, some kind of representation of a symbolic object, to focus and fix cross-modal representations. If that's so, then you don't need a more abstract representation – the cross-modal representation is abstract enough.

But these are questions that lie squarely within your territory, Bill, and I'd rather hear what you have to say about them.

WHC: The visual attributes of an apple are likely to reside near visual cortex, its auditory template is likely to be near auditory cortex, and the vocalization motor program needed to pronounce "apple" is likely to be in the rear of the frontal lobe. (That's the tentative conclusion from studying strokes, as when the color of an apple can be lost without the patient losing its characteristic shape or taste). So the full-fledged concept of an apple is not stored in some particular location; it's more like a distributed data base where a multifaceted report can be pulled together when needed.

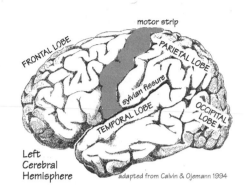

Left Cerebral Hemisphere

adapted from Calvin & Ojemann 1994

There are some major improvements that the human brain may have made, concerning how fast and flexibly the multi-modality linkups can be made. Let me save this issue until I've explained something about cortical circuitry.

Okay, we'll get back to it. But before we leave words and get on to sentences I'd like to comment on a recent suggestion that the rubicon between our species and others falls at the symbolic rather than the syntactic level. In other words, it's words, not sentences, that dramatically distinguish our species from others. Anyone who makes this kind of claim has to explain how it is that Sherman, Kanzi, and other trained apes have acquired symbolic representation to the extent – quite considerable – that they have. True, this level was attained only under human instruction, but because there are so many things we absolutely can't teach apes to do *at all*, we may reasonably conclude that no animal can learn things that fall outside its biological capacity – even if most animals can learn some things that their species doesn't usually do. So there remains the possibility that evolution will enlarge the behavioral envelopes of other species, and that any of a number of advanced animals might, millions of years hence, spontaneously acquire symbolic representations, just as human ancestors once did. The fact of our current uniqueness by no means entails that we shall always be unique.

In fact, as was apparent nearly two decades ago, the real rubicon, unpalatable though this may be to the philosophically minded, is syntax, not symbols.

SO WHAT IS A WORD, FINALLY? A word is the combination of a mental representation of something, which may or may not exist in the real world, with a mental representation of a set of symbols (phonetic, orthographic, manual). What you utter are not words, but only the phonological representations of words. What you write are not words, only the orthographic representations of words. What you sign, if you know one of the sign languages of the deaf, are not words but only signed representations of words. It's a convenient shorthand to speak of "the words I spoke," or "the words you wrote," one that in practice we would find it impossible to do without. But, in fact, words are much more abstract than that.

If all you did was to link these representations, all you would have would be a language of isolated words: Bread. Life. Oak tree. Silence. There would be meaning, but not a lot of it. To get anywhere serious, words have to be put together.

———————

WHC: The other problem that symbols have faced is that the categories to which they refer are rather fuzzy. Endless tales from animal behavior illustrate that categories may not be any more precise than they need to be (indeed, they're sometimes so crude that major mistakes can be made, as when some birds attack their own offspring that have strayed beyond the guano ring and attempt to return to their nest). Categories can be pretty ad hoc, often formed around a prototype of the class (the robin is a prototype bird; the penguin is an outlier, something that you can argue about).

Categories of one, such as proper names, are easy for us, but that's because our brains have some specializations for them in the front end of the temporal lobes, just in front of where the specializations for facial recognition are located. While social species need to remember individuals for dominance and reciprocal altruism reasons, human group size is much larger than in the other great ape species.

Which reminds me, Derek – even in a protolanguage sentence, the words come with some intrinsic

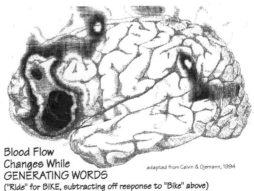

Blood Flow Changes While SPEAKING WORDS
(read aloud BIKE: "Bike," subtracting off response to reading it silently)

Blood Flow Changes While GENERATING WORDS   adapted from Calvin & Ojemann, 1994
("Ride" for BIKE, subtracting off response to "Bike" above)

information about possible roles. That's because of where nouns and verbs tend to be located in the brain. The temporal lobe is quite specialized for concepts (more later) used as nouns and adjectives, while the frontal lobe is probably the natural home for verbs and the relative orientation words such as "left," "before," "above," and so forth. And that's probably true for our pre-protolanguage ancestors as well: in all mammals, the frontal lobe is used to move and prepare for movements, so it isn't surprising to find verbs there, at least verbs for when you're the actor. But were you to stick your head into a brain scanner and try to find verbs that would go with a noun spoken to you (I say "bike," you reply, "Ride?"), much of the area above your left temple would probably light up (meaning that the inferior frontal lobe was requesting more blood flow because it was working harder).

Try to put together the simplest noun and verb for the first time, and you're probably invoking a long-distance circuit in the brain, a linkup between temporal and frontal lobes. Though, while looking down at the exposed brain surface during neurosurgery, they might seem within a few centimeters of one another, the route between them is actually more like the quickest land route between Spain and Morocco (via Israel!). Frontal and temporal lobes are connected by a very long loop through a white matter bundle called the arcuate fasciculus that detours around the huge infolding known as the insula. Just think of the temporal lobe as North Africa.

But because of this primitive, pre-protolanguage tagging of nouns and verbs by lobe of origin, you're not likely to mistake "William" for a verb, much as I've always aspired to write a memoir entitled *My Life As an Active Verb*. It does show you an aspect of language that segregates, though it's nothing at all like the performance-competence segregation that some expected from brain mapping.

3

Why Putting Words Together Isn't Easy

Now that we have a stock of words, we need to make sentences with them. My bet is, the first thing you'll think of in this connection is putting them into some sort of order. Indeed, there are even syntacticians who think that the most important thing about syntax is putting words into some kind of fixed order. By the time we get to the end of this chapter I hope to have convinced you that putting words into fixed orders is the least important part of structuring sentences – if indeed it's part of it at all.

The language acquisitionist Leila Gleitman once joked that when linguists talk about acquiring language, most of them explain how to get as far as "The cat sat on the mat" – and then they cross their fingers. Well, let's at least get to "The cat sat on the mat."

No problem. You have two nouns, a "cat" and a "mat," that refer to concrete objects. You have a verb, "sat," that refers to an action. You have a preposition "on," that tells you where something happened, and you have "the," which suggests that

> 'Only connect.'
> E.M. FORSTER

you ought to know which cat and which mat I'm talking about, without more ado. So you take the subject, whatever performs the action, and put it at the beginning, followed by the verb, followed by the location where the action of the verb took place. How else could you do it? It's dead easy, right?

Wrong. We are coming at this from our knowledge of English. But the human ancestors we are talking about didn't speak English. They didn't speak any kind of human language. A word-like "subject," even an abstract noun like "location," would have been far beyond their reach. Terms like "subject" and "object" can only be defined over a syntax that already exists. Before syntax existed, they were meaningless. For that matter, ancestral humans are very unlikely to have had words like "on" or "the."

What's an "on"? What's a "the"? These words don't correspond to anything in the observable universe. They're strictly relational. Even today, the first words of children don't include items like these, though they may well include nouns like "cat" and "mat," and even a verb or two. It's highly unlikely that our remote ancestors had more than a few nouns and verbs – at least not to start with. At best, then, they would have had "cat," and "mat," and "sat" (or more likely "sit," since past tense is a sophisticated feature of language).

Some languages (like Japanese and Turkish) are verb-final – "Cat mat sit." A lot of languages (German, for instance) are what is called "verb-second" languages, and in these you can have "Mat sit cat" just as easily as "Cat sit mat." A lot of Austronesian languages have the verb at the beginning ("Sit cat mat") while some also have the subject at the end ("Sit mat cat"). Literary Latin and some Australian languages just mix them up in any order at all, making use of inflections and role-specific words (as when we say "him" rather than "he") to convey roles.

All right, so word order is more of a problem than it might seem at first. However, given a speech community where everyone agreed on the meanings of "cat," "sit," and "mat," it would surely only be a matter of time before some kind of word order convention was agreed upon.

BUT THIS WOULDN'T SOLVE ALL THE PROBLEMS. And the most obvious of these problems is that there's no way you can be sure that all the elements of the sentence would be expressed. If someone thought you already had the cat in mind they might just say "sit mat" and assume you could figure out by yourself that they were talking about the cat. Same if they thought you knew about the mat – "cat sit" ought to do it, in that case. Or just "cat," or just "sit," or just "mat." Little kids of eighteen months or so seem to get on just fine with one-word sentences like these.

Those of us who are a little older might have problems with listening to a language that kept leaving you to figure out things for yourself all the time. When some people talk, it's hard enough to figure out what they really *mean* even when they put everything in – imagine what it would be like if they could leave out anything they liked, and you had to devote half your time and effort just to filling the gaps! The thing about real language is, you may have a hard time with the content, but the form of it, the way the sentences are actually put together, hardly ever gives you problems. You don't even notice it. It's like it was transparent. Your brain handles the form automatically (and perhaps that's why seeing the essential aspects of structure are so difficult for us).

But that automatic processing comes about only because there is syntax – principles and procedures for arranging words in ways such that long strings of words can be uttered effortlessly and understood equally effortlessly. Before you had syntax, all that existed was a kind of protolanguage.

IF YOU WANT TO KNOW what that protolanguage was like, you can get some idea by looking at the productions of apes who have been taught to use signs or other symbols, or at early-stage pidgin languages (at about the "Me Tarzan – you Jane" level of development), or at the speech of children under two. I say "get some idea," because of course there will be differences between then and now.

We can assume our early ancestors talked about more things than apes do and that some of those things were different from the things apes talk about. We know that speakers of any pidgin speak at least one natural human language fluently, and there has to be some carry-over (though if you look at samples of pidgin speech, it will amaze you to see how little), at least in the range of things that can be discussed. We know that children, especially if they are learning an inflected language like Spanish or Italian, will pick up the odd grammatical feature you won't find among apes or early stage pidgin speakers, and probably wouldn't have found among our remote ancestors, either. All protolanguage varieties:

> ▷ can only string together a small handful of words at a time;
> ▷ can leave out any words they feel like leaving out;
> ▷ often depart from the customary word order unpredictably and for no obvious reason;
> ▷ cannot form any complex structures, whether these be complex noun phrases or sentences more than a clause long;
> ▷ contain, if they have any at all, only a tiny fraction of the inflections and the "grammatical words" – things such as articles, prepositions and the like – that make up 50 percent of true language utterances.

Now the question is, why are these protolanguage varieties – ape-talk, toddler talk, pidgin – the way they are?

LET'S ASSUME THAT YOU HAVE WORDS and that you've somehow managed to sort out a convention about word order, so that everyone says "John kissed Mary" (as we do in English) rather than "John Mary kissed," as they would in Japanese. Surely, once you had gotten that far, you could very easily just go on building longer and longer sentences until gradually, over time, language attained the complexity it has today. Wrong.

There are lots of reasons why that doesn't work. First, let's suppose that you didn't want to say, "John kissed Mary." You want to say "That boy kissed Mary," but when you say it you see from my look that I don't know which boy you mean, so you say "That boy you saw yesterday kissed Mary." Something's wrong here. Sentences start with a noun and follow it with a verb, but here there are two nouns (well, a noun and a pronoun, "boy" and "you") together before you even get to a verb, and they seem to refer to different people, like in the "John Mary kissed" Japanese-style sentence above.

What's happened to our word order convention? Shouldn't this new sentence start with "That boy saw you"? But in that case, "you" would come before "kissed Mary," and I know I didn't kiss Mary yesterday or ever. Could "saw" maybe be a noun? No, because then you'd have three nouns in a row instead of two. But then you've got "yesterday kissed Mary." Come on. Days can't kiss people, only people can kiss people. Just what kind of nonsense is this, anyway?

There would be no reason for anyone hearing this sentence to suppose that the whole string, "That boy you saw," is in fact the subject, while "kissed Mary" is simply its predicate. In fact, at the stage of language development we're talking about, nobody would have had the faintest idea what a subject or a predicate was. Indeed, I'm cheating a bit even in just imagining some cave-dwelling ancestor sweating bullets while struggling to understand such sentences, because nobody back then could have produced them. Moreover, since comprehension usually runs well ahead of production (think of Kanzi the bonobo, or of yourself struggling with high-school Spanish or German), you would find those sentences even harder to produce than to understand.

THE REASON FOR THIS IS AS FOLLOWS. A simple grammar like we've envisaged – a grammar with a fixed order in which subject precedes predicate and the verb of the predicate, if transitive, precedes its object – works just fine, so long as all you have are nouns and verbs and no more than one verb per utterance. Then you can parse easily: first word, a noun, so the subject; second word, a verb, head of the predicate; third word, a noun, therefore the other half of the predicate. So here's a grammar, you may think, that would at least give you "John kissed Mary" or "The cat sat on the mat" (as it might, but for the zinger that's waiting in the wings).

But it only works as long as you stick to single words, single nouns and verbs. Once you get a complex structure as your topic (like "That boy you saw yesterday"), you're in trouble – because you don't know, and you have nothing that will help you find out, where the units in the sentence begin and end. You might manage "that boy," because there's no other noun involved, but once you get to "boy you," you're lost. All your experience tells you two nouns mean two referents (and they do) but your grammar tells you that no two nouns can come together in this way.

Indeed, whenever we find an example of protolanguage, whether it be child speech, pidgin, or an ape's attempts at language, we find that it consists of nouns and verbs without modifiers of any kind (except for very occasional common adverbs or adjectives, often incorporated into a single, rote-learned phrase). It's worth noting that apes haven't gotten past this stage, children nearly always do, and a few adult pidgin speakers may succeed (although the vast majority do not).

It looks like we are in the presence of something that is specific to the human species but that children do much better than adults – sure signs of a biological property with the kind of window of opportunity known as a "critical period" (if the property doesn't develop before the period's over, it may never do so).

WHC: That reminds me of our discussion back when we first got to Bellagio (p. 10). Children are enormously acquisitive of patterns, starting with the infant's listening to language during its first year and devising categories for the common speech sounds (about forty phonemes in English); at six months, a Japanese infant can still hear the difference between the English /L/ and /R/ but, by age one, he or she no longer hears the difference, with a nearby Japanese phoneme capturing all nearby speech sounds as mere variants, standardizing them. "Rice" and "lice" would sound the same.

Then the baby starts acquiring combinations of phonemes, i.e., words, at the rate of about nine new words every day. Somewhere between 18 and 36 months of age, children figure out the common patterns of words in sentences, and make a fairly fast transition into speaking with phrases and clauses. They aren't taught rules. (What parent could possibly explain them? Especially in babytalk?) Instead, they guess the underlying structure, from what they hear. So far as I can see, they go on to discover narrative structure and then start criticizing bedtime stories that lack proper endings.

Four major phases of acquisitiveness, each building upon the one before – and even by children of modest intelligence. Deaf children surrounded by fluent sign language (from deaf parents, deaf babysitters, or deaf preschool) make a parallel set of discoveries – but they don't do very well if deprived of such opportunities until school age; the preschool years are the natural time for such discoveries, and "making up for it" later between the ages of seven and fifteen is increasingly ineffective. That's the prime evidence for a "critical period" in language development, along with the tragic stories of abused children locked away from opportunities to hear speech and their frequent failures to subsequently acquire language fluency.

So, is there an "epigenetic rule" that says "Seek structure amid chaos"? Is that what chimps and bonobos lack, or do they lack syntax wiring? (Or both?) To form a new category, such as the notion of a prepositional phrase, might require a lot of varied examples of it, before seeing the regularities of structure in the input. If reared in an environment that lacks a lot of examples of such structures (say, dozens within a week's time), it might be difficult to zero in on it. So-called "fast mapping" says that it requires dozens of exposures to a new word (not just one, at least when it is embedded in a complex environment with lots of other things going on) before learning it; the same might be the case for syntax and narrative structures.

IF ALL THERE WAS was an "epigenetic rule" that said "Seek structure amid chaos," there would be no creole languages. Creole languages come into existence when parents who speak a structureless early-stage pidgin pass it on to their children. The children change that pidgin, in a single generation, into a full-fledged language. If they were seeking structure in the pidgin, they wouldn't find any – they impose structure from within their own minds), Rather than acquiring a vague general capacity to "seek structure" – how would any creature do that? – I think we acquired the capacity to create structure in language and that capacity then generalized to apply in other spheres.

WHC: But "seek structure amid chaos" allows for guessing wrong, finding structure in the environment when there is none.

We fool ourselves all the time. (Think of astrology!) It isn't much of a further step to invention without a model, so long as those Universal Grammar circuitry underpinnings are really there to guide the invention. Epigenetic tendencies (like "seek structure") and innate circuitry (like UG's resonances) are two separate things, though surely they have co-evolved somewhat.

Naturally. We, like most other creatures, are built to make generalizations on inadequate evidence at very short notice, because that works better, in terms of evolutionary fitness, than making 100 percent correct generalization after a long period of cogitation. But other creatures don't have language, so there's no way the "language instinct" could be "seeking structure" and nothing more. Besides, that leaves unanswered the question of why, out of the zillions of kinds of structure that it could have, language just has the one it does.

Anyway, we can be pretty sure that no creature without the appropriate internal structure can learn to increase the size of a descriptive phrase. We can. We can go from "hats" to "black hats," to "three black hats," to "those three black hats," to "those three black hats with brims," to "those three black hats with broad brims," to "those three black hats with broad brims that remind you of the hats the bad guys in late-night Western movies wear," and any of these would fit the empty slot in "I'd like to buy____" or "____would look good on you." The reason is not because speakers of a protolanguage cannot add one word to another – they surely can. What they can't do is know where to stop, where the boundaries lie between one descriptive phrase and another. And the reason for this is that, in protolanguage, there are no units of intermediate size between the single word and the entire utterance. In other words, there are no such things as phrases and clauses. Without phrases and clauses we can't establish boundaries within the utterance, and as a result of this we become victims of ever increasing ambiguity.

We saw ambiguities and plain old-fashioned confusions arising in plenty out of the attempt by a protolanguage speaker to parse "That boy you saw yesterday kissed Mary." But suppose the sentence was "That boy you saw kissed the girl he liked." Still only nine words, but to the previous ambiguities would now be added the following: Is the last part another misconstructed subject-predicate (really "the girl liked him"), or is "kissed the girl" a complete predicate — in which case what do we do with "he liked"? Liked what? If what he liked was "the girl," why not say so? Note too that these ambiguities can't be resolved in isolation. Because they arise from not knowing where the boundaries are (or rather from simply not having boundaries at all), each possible parse of each segment increases the possible parses of the whole utterance exponentially. One ambiguity gives two possible readings, two ambiguities give four, three give eight, and so on. Very soon, as you see, the ambiguities become too numerous for anyone to cope with, which is one reason why protolanguage utterances are almost always confined to four or five words at most — and usually less.

BUT THIS STILL ISN'T THE WORST. I said there was a factor that would quickly destabilize any attempt to give structure to language by providing it with a rigid word order; in fact, it's already been referred to, briefly, in this chapter. It's this: Sure, you can say "John kissed Mary," and we have agreed that, by convention, possible alternatives — "John Mary kissed," "kissed John Mary" — would eventually be ruled out. But in protolanguage nothing tells you that you have to say *all* of "John kissed Mary" — that you have, obligatorily, to put in a word describing the action and two others describing the two actors.

Now you may argue that the same is true of our language. If you ask "Who did John kiss?" I don't (outside of an English as a foreign language class!) have to say "John kissed Mary." It's much more natural if I just say "Mary." Similarly, if you ask "Who kissed Mary," I would answer simply, "John," or "John did." If you asked "What did John and Mary do when they met," I could say, "They kissed," or just "Kissed." But that's only true in the context of answering direct questions. In any other context, if I were to say "John kissed," or "kissed Mary," or simply "kissed," you would immediately feel something was missing and blame me for not telling you who kissed and/or who got kissed, even if you already knew those things. It's true, a boxing referee may say "Break," or a surgeon may say "Forceps," but because we all know a full human language, and because we know something about the conventions of boxing rings and operating theaters, we know that the first remark is just shorthand for "You two better break your clinch" and the second for "Pass me the forceps, please." We understand such remarks because they stand against the background of a language where, in the vast majority of cases, certain things have to be stated fully.

But before there was such a language – and obviously language like we have today could not have sprung up fully formed from the beginning – then there was no way in which we could have known what *had* to be said or even that there were things that had to be said. We had words and that was all. We could use as few or as many as were wanted, limited only by our power to utter them and the hearer's power to understand them. As practitioners of a behavior that had barely begun, the natural inclination would have been – as it still is in the contemporary forms of protolanguage – to say as little as we could get away with. It's less effort to say things like "John kissed" and "kissed Mary" than to say "John kissed Mary." The less you say, the less chance there is that you will make a mistake or a fool of yourself, and if there is enough previous knowledge and/or situational context, hearers may be able to figure out for themselves who got kissed or did the kissing.

WHC: And I provided a good example the other day, in trying to communicate with the Villa waiter whose English is limited. "Don't say too much," was Susan Sontag's writerly advice from across the breakfast table. If I stuck to several English nouns, the waiter could guess my meaning; in trying to speak a real sentence, I was just confusing the waiter, who didn't know English syntax well enough to parse more words. Maybe the language-reared apes, in sticking to short utterance lengths, are just practicing Sontag's advice: saying just enough to allow us to guess their intention, their mental model underlying the attempted communication.

THIS FREEDOM TO SAY ANYTHING OR NOTHING, this free-for-all that's inescapable in any communication system without rules or structure, simply compounds the already more than sufficiently compounded ambiguities that beset every protolanguage utterance. And if by this time you are thoroughly confused, like the centipede who started to wonder which foot he put down first – completely unable to understand how on earth you can produce the simplest sentence – that's fine. That's how I want you to be. Because that's how anyone should be, faced with the awesome mystery of how anything as seemingly complex as language could ever have bootstrapped itself into existence – yet still be learnable by children who can't tie their shoelaces or use a spoon without spilling its contents all over themselves. And it's nothing to do with being smart. Children with a condition known as Williams' Syndrome with IQs of 40 or 50 can run together sentences just as well as you or I. What they say may be false or silly, but the way it's put together is impeccable. Language is an awesome mystery, and we'll get nowhere by pretending that it isn't.

So now we've got some conception of the difficulty of the task of producing even fairly simple sentences, a task that has so far defeated all species but our own. Now we can get down to examining the problem of how language evolved. Basically it's an engineering problem. We have to find some way of providing structural units intermediate between the word and the complete utterance. Given the appropriate units (such as phrases and clauses), we should be able to perform all the complex computations that human language requires. But those units must have come from somewhere – we couldn't have simply invented them. So the units, whatever they are, need a plausible history, in addition to an explanation of how, exactly, they make language possible.

WHC: I like that statement of the problem, because it allows for something else besides the obvious usefulness-for-language to provide some of the underlying structural tendencies. It's long been obvious to neuroscientists that language function was likely to be mixed up, location-wise, with some other functions – that "language cortex" isn't *only* doing language tasks. There is an enormous overlap with oral-facial and hand-arm sequencing, for example, suggesting that improvements in one might have benefitted the others, at least at some stage in hominid evolution.

It also makes me wonder if what the language-reared apes are lacking, thus far, is simply a good sense of phrase boundaries – which could be accomplished by a sensitivity to boundary words like "and" and "into." There aren't very many of them, just a few dozen, and apes might be able to learn them as special words that signal a new phrase or clause. So far, the attempts to teach apes the "closed-class words" have been minor, though I'm told they're on the agenda for the next round of work with language-reared bonobos.

DB: Bill, the problem isn't that simple. I agree it will be fun to try and teach bonobos boundary words. In fact, I just learned from my old friend and colleague Talmy Givon that he has submitted a proposal to do just that. Lack of the right words is part of the problem, but by no means all of it. Where are the boundary markers in "That boy you saw yesterday kissed Mary" or "The boy you saw kissed the girl he liked"? Thinking that you get the boundaries from the boundary markers just puts things back to front – you have to get the boundaries first and then put in the markers. And that's not happenstance. It has to be that way, because until you know what the boundaries bound, you can't know how to correctly use the markers. But there'll be more on this in a chapter or two.

WHC: Kanzi (a bonobo, or pygmy chimpanzee, with more than a decade of language tutoring) can comprehend novel, never heard before, sentences as complex as "Kanzi, go to the office and bring back the red ball." He makes about as many mistakes as a two-and-a-half-year-old child does, on the same tests of interpreting novel requests. Of course, the child goes on to produce such sentences, and Kanzi is still stuck back at the stage of two-word requests, with an occasional third word.

Linguists, I know, are impressed only by production abilities (as it is instantly apparent whether or not the speaker knows how to unambiguously structure a long utterance). But, in some sense, understanding is said to be the harder task, because you have to correctly guess the speaker's state of mind; in production, you know your state of mind and "merely" have to get it across to another. Once sentences start to lengthen and possibilities for ambiguity develop, production becomes difficult without knowing how to structure a sentence.

Maybe it's just my motor systems physiology background talking (thought as preparation for action, seeking additional sensory input to help decide between alternative possibilities for one's next act), but I tend to be impressed by performance, including Kanzi's ability to carry out a complicated series of instructions for the first time, and get it right. That shows us that bonobos have got the brains for understanding requests of some complexity, even to the extent of some phrases within the sentence. To produce such sentences himself, Kanzi would need to craft a novel request in such a way that there is little ambiguity. Appreciating someone else's potential confusion (one of the fancier aspects of a "theory of mind") is certainly important for serious writers, but language learners likely have acquired simpler conventions for structuring long utterances.

DB: Bill, I'm afraid we'll have to agree to disagree here. Production is harder than comprehension, as anyone knows who has attempted to learn a foreign language. The fabled difficulties of understanding are exaggerated. In the first place, some of those difficulties exist only for overcerebralized Western academics — most folks have no trouble reading others' states of mind via body language and horse sense. In the second, we must distinguish between what something means and what somebody means by it.

If I say, "Gee, it's cold in here!" you may not know whether I am making a factual remark, or want you to light a fire, or hope to persuade you to move elsewhere. However, you have no trouble in deciding what the words themselves mean — they mean that it's damn cold in here, and my state of mind has nothing to do with that. I doubt whether, in the case you mention, Kanzi needed to know anything about the state of Sue Savage-Rumbaugh's mind.

In fact, in understanding what something means, we have all sorts of clues from semantics, pragmatics, and situational context that are quite useless when it comes to production. I don't think for a moment that Kanzi knew the grammatical structure of "Go to the office and bring back the red ball" – if he knew what "go," "office," "bring," and "red ball" meant, he wouldn't have to be the bonobo equivalent of a rocket scientist to figure out what he had to do. And if he did understand the grammatical structure, what's stopping him from producing sentences like this himself?

4

Bigger than a Word,
Smaller than a Sentence

What are the basic differences between protolanguage and real language? Let's look at one property of the stringing words together process that produces protolanguage. I pointed out a while back that protolanguage characteristically consists almost exclusively of nouns and verbs, without any modifiers – if adverbs appear, they are usually whole-utterance modifiers, not modifiers of single words. If adjectives appear, they are a few of the more common ones, probably acquired with nouns as unanalyzed chunks, like idioms. But what this means is that all units are of equal value, just as you would expect them to be if they are all hung on the same clothesline.

Put it another way. In protolanguage, all words are equal; like runners in a race, it's every word for itself. But if protolanguage is a footrace, language is a team sport, like football. The teams are phrases, and like any team, not all the players are equal – there's a captain, and there are just regular players. In language we call these "heads" and "modifiers." You can always tell what the head is by asking what the phrase is about. Is the phrase "a young teacher of algebra from Oklahoma" about a teacher, algebra, or Oklahoma? A teacher, obviously – all the other words modify the word "teacher."

The way we diagram sentences reflects this. Take "John kissed Mary." This could be either a true-language sentence or a protolanguage utterance. Don't get the idea that protolanguage has to consist entirely of mangled utterances like "John kissed" or "kissed Mary." It will probably contain a majority of these, but there's nothing to prevent something that looks like a proper sentence from popping out now and then (though likely missing that -*ed* for past tense). The only difference, for reasons we'll get to in a moment, is that it will sound like "John...kissed...Mary" rather than "JohnkissedMary."

So this is how "John kissed Mary" gets put together in the two modes:

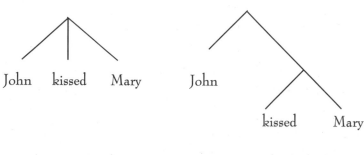

PROTOLANGUAGE   LANGUAGE with syntax

Now if they made you do this sort of thing in school you may well be thinking, "These are just drawings, they don't have anything to do with how sentences are produced." But I think that's wrong. I think that these diagrams really show you what happens in the brain. If the brain is working in protolanguage mode, each word is sent separately to the part of the brain that controls the motor organs of speech, and each word is uttered separately.

When I first arrived in Hawaii, back in 1972, one of the things that struck me most forcibly was the difference in speed between the old-time immigrants who'd come to the island as young adults and spoke pidgin, and their children, born in Hawaii, who spoke creole (which in Hawaii is also called "pidgin," just to confuse things a bit more!). On top of all the other differences in their speech, the old-timers spoke about three times slower than their own kids. For instance, here's an old-timer trying to describe one of those clock/thermometers you often see on the sides of city buildings:

"Building – high place – wall part – time – now-time – and then – now temperature every time give you."

If you've ever been in foreign country where you spoke only a few words of the language, you'll know how it feels to speak protolanguage – anguished search for a word, struggle to pronounce it, anguished search for the next word, and so on.

WHC· My Italian is at this level of protolanguage. My Italian comprehension is no better that Kanzi's understanding of English, and my utterance lengths in Italian are no better than Kanzi's either! Yet most linguists would classify my Italian as "language" understanding and production, even though they hesitate to classify Kanzi's as such. It's still a dual standard, even though the accomplishments of the language-reared apes have become so impressive.

Absolutely. But if the brain is working in language mode, words are put together in whole phrases and clauses and even sentences before they're sent to the speech organs to be pronounced. That's why, when you're speaking your own native language, the words come out like a blue streak.

The second diagram illustrates another important fact. If you take it from the bottom up, rather than the top down, it reflects not just *the fact that* but *the order in which* the brain puts words together. That is to say, "kissed" and "Mary" are joined, before "John" is joined to "kissed Mary."

Which brings us to parsing.

THE WORD "PARSE" has come in for some pretty vicious abuse lately. As a result of Clinton's impeachment trial, people talk about speakers "parsing" words like "sex" or "alone" in the sense of determining, sometimes quite arbitrarily, how those words should be interpreted. This usage is daft in two ways. First, you can't parse single *words* – you can only parse *sentences*. Second, parsing isn't something speakers do, it's

something hearers do. A hearer parses a sentence (quite unconsciously —
unless it's in a syntax class!) by deciding what that sentence's structure is.

Of course, that's not quite the whole story. If I say "Would you mind
stopping that noise?" you don't respond by thinking, "Ah! An auxiliary verb
followed by a second-person pronoun subject of the main verb 'mind,' followed in turn by a
participial verb that takes a noun-phrase consisting of noun and determiner for its object,"
and leave it at that. You parse sentences to find out their meaning. You
need to know that I am speaking to you, that I want you to do something,
and what it is that I want you to do. I suppose it's this rather indirect
link with meaning that folk have taken as license to abuse the poor word.

Anyway, parsing is something we all do every time anything is uttered.
But it works quite differently depending on whether what's uttered is
language or protolanguage. In fact, if it's protolanguage, it's a good
question whether you can be said to parse at all. You can't decide what
the structure is if there isn't any structure. What you do is just the
second part of the job, trying to determine the meaning directly from the
individual words. This of course is much harder than it is when there's
structure there to help you. You have to use all your knowledge of who's
speaking and what's happening and what the world in general is like in
order to figure out what is meant.

Suppose you hear a protolanguage utterance like "John kissed." You
might think, that's easy — all I have to do is figure out who John is most
likely to have kissed. But suppose the speaker is a pidgin speaker from
Japan. It's possible in that case that the meaning is, "somebody kissed John,"
because verbs come at the end of the sentence in Japanese, and pidgin
speakers sometimes (but pretty unpredictably) carry over features of their
native languages into their pidgin. This is just one of the many reasons
you can't hope to interpret protolanguage without taking lots of context
into account (and doing plenty of guesswork, too).

Now take an actual headline I saw in the *Denver Post* the other day:
"Spy Charges Dog Inspectors." You can't understand this sentence unless you
get the structure right, and know that "Charges" is here a noun, not a verb;
that "Spy Charges" is a subject; and that "Dog" is a verb. Of course you
may have first spotted an alternative parse: "Spy" as subject, "Charges" as

verb, "Dog Inspectors" as object. If you don't get the structure, you can't get the right meaning.

Here you may reasonably object, "Well, you need context just as much here. If you didn't know that the story under the headline concerned weapons inspectors in Iraq, you might assume that some spy had leveled unspecified charges against people whose job it was to inspect dogs, or had made them pay him some money." That's perfectly true; the headline had me baffled until I looked at the text. But two things make this case very different.

First, you very seldom need context to get the meaning of a true-language utterance, whereas you almost always need context to get the meaning of a protolanguage utterance (when I reread transcripts of pidgin speakers that I myself have recorded and transcribed, I often have no idea what they're talking about, although I can remember they made perfect sense at the time). Second, and much more important, you're using context in quite different ways. With the headline, you're using context to choose between two equally grammatical structures; with proto-language, you're using context to try and get any meaning at all.

This particular contrast between language and protolanguage shows up best when you look at what linguists call "empty categories." An empty category is where some unit of a sentence isn't overtly expressed. Take a sentence like "Bill wanted to go." "Wanted" has an overt subject but "go" doesn't have an overt subject, though we know that it must have a subject, and that its subject must be "Bill." Empty categories are rather like protons. You can't see any protons in this page you're reading, but you know they're there because your physics teacher told you so. Your English teacher should have told you the same thing about "missing" subjects and objects, but probably didn't (even though to me they're among the most fascinating things about language, I'm not going to force them on you here; if you choose, you can read more about them in the appendix on page 227, 230).

Again, there's a superficial resemblance between language and protolanguage that masks a profound difference. Protolanguage too has "missing" things, such as a missing subject in "kissed Mary" and a missing object in "John kissed." But the antecedents of these empty categories – the people or things they refer to – can't be found anywhere in the utterance. To know what those missing items refer to, you have to take into account who and what you're talking about and, on that basis and your general knowledge, you have to work out who or what the speaker is most likely to be talking about. In real language, the antecedent is always there somewhere in the sentence, and there are rules to help you find it.

You can read more about those rules in the appendix. Enough for now to note that you can't just assume that the nearest noun is the antecedent of the empty category. That's true in "Bill wanted to go" and "Bill wanted Helen to go," but not in "Helen was the one that Bill wanted to go." In both the last two sentences, "Helen" is the subject of "go," but in the first she's next to the verb and in the second she's far from it and "Bill" is much nearer. The rules that fix the reference of empty categories are not simple, not obvious, and above all, not consciously applied. You just somehow know that, despite the distance between "Helen" and "go," it's her that, hopefully, will do the going.

Now we come to what's maybe the most crucial difference between language and protolanguage: the existence in the former of phrases and clauses that are entirely absent from the latter. Such intermediate units cause problems. For instance, how are we going to tell where they begin or end?

THERE'S A SIMPLE ANSWER to this that, like most simple answers, doesn't give you the whole story. You might say, "When you come to the end of what a phrase is about, and start a phrase about something else, you know you've crossed a boundary." That's easy in

The pink shirt is dirty.

It's less easy in

The pink shirt you made me buy is dirty.

and even more so in

The pink shirt you made me buy when we stopped off
on the way to Cincinnati is dirty.

The trouble is, a phrase can be indefinitely long, and can include any number of things that might seem, to an outside observer, to have nothing to do with whatever is the head of the phrase.

The only way you can know where things begin and end is by knowing what phrases and clauses are. And, unfortunately for the common-sense, gradual-evolutionist view that maybe first phrases developed, then clauses (or vice versa), the two can only be defined in terms of one another (a phrase without a clause makes almost as little sense as a clause without a phrase):

> A **phrase** is a group of words making up a participant in the state, process or action expressed by a clause.
>
> A **clause** is a group consisting of a verb and all the phrases that express participants in its state, process or action.

WHC: Ah, verbs. When I was teaching myself to read scientific French and German, they were the key to survival. Find all the verbs in the sentence, I thought, and the structure of the rest would fall into place. If there was ambiguity remaining, I'd go in search of the prepositions. Unfortunately, this principle did not suffice for spoken language, where elements were often missing and had to be inferred.

DB: Naturally, but I bet verbs were never missing – that can only happen in protolanguage.

What this means is that a clause is a clause because it has the right number of phrases ("Fred put his new credit card into his wallet," rather than "Fred put his new credit card," where there is a phrase too few, or "Fred put his sister his new credit card into his wallet." where there is one too many). And a phrase is a phrase because it expresses a participant in the action of the verb and because it occupies a particular position in a clause (say, between the verb and "into his wallet" for "his new credit card." And the two are even more entangled than that. A phrase can contain a clause, which in turn includes phrases of its own, as in

The pink shirt that you made me buy is dirty.

where "The pink shirt that you made me buy" contains the clause "(that) you made me buy," and where this clause, in turn, contains several phrases (to syntacticians, "you" and "me" are just as much phrases as "The pink shirt" or "The tall blond man with one black shoe" — a phrase is anything that has a head, regardless of whether that head has any modifiers). The fact that these two units, intermediate between word and sentence, can operate in this way is what gives language one of its most striking characteristics, its infinite recursivity.

In his book *The Language Instinct*, Steven Pinker refers to what the *Guinness Book of Records* claimed as the longest English sentence: a 1,300-word monster by William Faulkner beginning "They both bore it as though in deliberate flagellant exaltation . . ." Pinker correctly pointed out that he could break that record by simply writing *"Faulkner wrote, 'They both bore it as though in deliberate flagellant exaltation . . .'"*

What's happening here is that Pinker is converting Faulkner's 1,300 word monster into a mere phrase, a noun-phrase object whose function is no different from that of "a book" in "Faulkner wrote a book." And as Pinker points out, anyone with ambitions to get into the Guinness Book could do so by adding "Pinker wrote that Faulkner wrote . . ." or "Who cares that Pinker wrote that Faulkner wrote . . ." The process is truly an infinite one, limited only by our shortish immediate memories and the difficulty of making infinite sense.

BUT WHERE DID PHRASES AND CLAUSES COME FROM? If they're as closely interlinked as I've suggested, how can one be the hen and the other the egg? All we've seen so far suggests that they were born as twins, and that some third thing has to underlie both phrases and clauses. And indeed it does. That thing is what is known as "argument structure."

When you get down to it, the basic task of language is telling you who did what to whom (as well as when, where, how, and occasionally why). These "WH-words," as linguists call them (although "how" has its W at the wrong end), just about exhaust the questions you can ask – even in plain old "Yes-No" questions, you're asking WHether something happened or not. We can conclude from this that there's a limit to the number of participants there can be in any action, process or state. Or at least that there's a limit to the number we can talk about. We can talk about who performed an action, or who underwent it, or to whom it was directed, or for whose benefit it was performed, or when, where, or how it was performed.

But there's no way we can talk *directly* about who observed it, or who discussed it. If I say "Bill kicked the cat," you know without more ado that Bill performed the action and the cat underwent it. But there's no way I can say anything like "Bill kicked the cat blik me," meaning "Bill kicked the cat observed by me," or "Bill kicked the cat plok us," meaning "Bill kicked the cat discussed by us." Things like that can of course be expressed – you can express anything in language, given time, patience, and ingenuity – but they have to be expressed indirectly: "I observed Bill kicking the cat" or "We discussed the fact that Bill had kicked the cat." In other words, we have to downgrade the original sentence into some kind of phrase or clause, then insert it into another clause.

Now you'll have noticed that each of the participants in these states or actions has a specific role to play. There are AGENTS that perform actions, PATIENTS or THEMES that undergo them, GOALS to which they are directed, and so on. These roles are known as "thematic roles." A thematic role plus the noun-phrase ,to which that role is attached, make up what is known as an "argument." And argument structure – the system that determines when and where arguments can appear in language – represents the crucial link between word meaning (semantics) and sentence structure (syntax). Not every syntactician would make argument structure central to an account of syntax as it is today. But that's irrelevant. How something started is often very different to what it has become – for instance, try describing modern computers in the terms appropriate for their ancestors of just forty or fifty years ago.

BEFORE THERE WAS SYNTAX, there was only semantics. So, if you are looking for the very first stages in the development of syntax, you have to look in semantics for whatever is the most syntaxlike thing. Argument structure is the most plausible candidate. It involves meaning (the meanings of the thematic roles, AGENT and so on, and their relation to the verb meaning) but it can be readily mapped onto linguistic output to provide that output with structure, along the lines described below.

The first thing to note is that all arguments aren't equal. Some make an obligatory appearance, others only an optional one. It's as if a team had a small core of seasoned players that appeared predictably while the remainder sat in a bench awaiting a call. For instance, if you use the verb "kick," you are obliged to mention a kicker and a kickee. You're not obliged to mention where the kicking was done, or how, or when, or for whom (even if it was done on behalf of someone else), although of course you can whenever you need to. Likewise, if you use the verb "sleep," all you need do is name who slept – you don't need to say who was slept with, or for how long the person slept. That is to say, every verb demands that a certain number (not less than one, not more than three) of the participants *must* be expressed.

Is the fact that verbs are divided into three classes (on the basis of the number of arguments that obligatorily accompany them) a fact of nature or an artifact of analysis? Do all states, processes, and actions in the world fall into one of these groups because of the nature of reality, or does the structure of the human mind impose its own pattern? This is a philosophical issue and fortunately I don't think we need answer it here. You can be sure, whatever human language you may meet, that the verb equivalent to the English "sleep" will take one obligatory argument, the verb equivalent to "break" will take two, and the verb equivalent to "give" will require three.

You've heard about "false friends" in language learning: words that sound like words in your language but mean something quite different in the other. Well, the division of verbs into three argument classes is a true friend, and like all true friends, seldom fully appreciated and too often taken for granted.

But the importance of argument structure goes far beyond that. If you know that

> ▷ there are *phrases and clauses*, and you know that
> ▷ *clauses consist of verbs and their arguments*, and you know
> ▷ *how many arguments each verb must take*, and
> ▷ *what the thematic roles of those arguments are*,

then you can easily process sentences that would have had you buffaloed if all you had was protolanguage. Take for example a sentence we looked at in the previous chapter: "The boy you saw kissed the girl he liked." Parsing this with the above in mind, we look immediately at the verb "kissed" and know that it must take two arguments. Because the language is English, and because we know the way English maps argument structure onto phrase structure, we know that "kissed" will be followed by a THEME (whoever got kissed) and preceded by an AGENT (whoever did the kissing). But this isn't a simple "X kissed Y," because there are two extra verbs, "saw" and "liked," which should have their own arguments. So you look for these.

Start with "liked." That takes two obligatory arguments, but there's only one there. However, you know that the other *must* be there, somewhere, even if you can't see it, because the nature of argument structure tells you so. For every invisible argument there's a visible argument in the same sentence that refers to the same person or thing. Often (see the appendix for a more detailed treatment) you'll find that visible argument immediately next to the left of the leftmost obligatory argument of the verb you're working on: in this case, "the girl."

Now you turn to the first part of the sentence. Here, again, the verb "saw" should have two arguments but has only one, "you." Again you know it must be there, and must be linked in reference to the argument on the left of the leftmost argument of "saw" ("you"). That argument is "the boy."

You have successfully parsed "The boy you saw kissed the girl he liked," finding that it contains one main clause and two subordinate clauses modifying the heads "boy" and "girl." And in so doing you have arrived at its correct meaning – which of course is what the whole exercise is about. It's easy for people who work on syntax to get wrapped up in it and think that maybe it's not just everything, it's the only thing. Of course it's not. It's a mechanism, a means to an end, what allows you to move on to the next task.

But without that means, there wouldn't be an end. Syntax is the magic key that unlocks the floodgates of language, unleashes the irresistible torrent of words that has swept us to where we are today. But where did that key come from, and how did we come by it?

LET ME BRIEFLY SUM UP WHERE WE'RE AT RIGHT NOW. I've just said that the core of syntax must contain the means for producing phrases and clauses, because these are the indispensable units intermediate between word and complete utterance. These units are indispensable because without them we could not produce true sentences, or indeed any kind of long and/or complex utterance that could be understood. Now phrases and clauses derive from argument structure – from the fact that verbs can only assign a limited number of arguments, and that every verb falls into one of three classes that assign one, two, or three obligatory arguments. respectively.

Naturally you'll want to know where argument structure came from and how we came to fashion our utterances in the ways that argument structure dictated. But before I can get to that, we'll need to look at what goes on in the brain when we use language.

So, over to you, Bill.

WHC: From *what* (words to syntax) and *why* (evolutionary) considerations, it's apparent that we need to know a lot more about *how* brains categorize an entity or a state of affairs, how this memory is retrieved and linked to others, and how we cope with the inevitable ambiguities. Both emergents (like crystals) and conversions of function (like curb cuts) could, at different times, be part of the story.

We're most accustomed to noun attributes (Derek's fruit with a color attribute, a shape attribute, the sound it makes when falling off the tree, and so forth). But they're all optional–you'll forgive me if I mention an apple without telling you its color or size. Verbs too have optional attributes, such as time and place, but each verb has one or more obligatory attributes. How that's implemented in the brain is surely a key question.

If I say (as the billboard ads have taken to doing) "Give him," you'll go looking for three noun phrases. You will happily infer that it's an imperative construction and supply the missing "you," but the lack of a noun for the THEME will disturb you, and you'll search for what you missed (supplied, in the ad, by a picture or logo). It's a technique for grabbing people skimming over the ad and bringing them to a screeching halt, making them pay attention, thanks to a subconscious process that rings alarm bells. We talk of computers "hanging up," and this is a prime example of a hung psychological process that might give us some clues to the circuitry someday.

By this point, I'm certainly curious about how the brain can do all of this, what circuits constitute the algorithm. I'm not sure that I can fully answer it (please don't ask me where the Empty Categories are located!), but let me creep up on the problem of brain circuits for structuring sentences by introducing language and memory circuits, Darwinian processes, and the brain's long-distance problem. Then we'll be able to speculate more intelligently about what neural machinery might have been co-opted for syntax.

5

Language in the Brain

Derek,

Well, I wasn't able to cover very much about the brain as comments on your language chapters, so let me try more systematically. Here's my short version of where mental abilities arise in the brain, strongly influenced by my varied dinner-table attempts to cover the subject for the others. This time, I'll do large scale features first, then zoom down to the cellular level of organization and slowly zoom back out – at least as far as the level associated with ensembles of neurons, which is where I think the big improvements occurred, the ones that enabled syntax to flourish.

Bill

L anguage is located in the brain, but you'd never guess where just from studying monkeys. As I mentioned in the context of aphasic patients who could still swear like sailors, exclamations seem to survive when the usual lateral language areas (just above, and in front of, your left ear) are damaged. Only damage to a rather distant area of cortex, in the midline above the corpus callosum, affects exclamations as well – and that's about where the cortical aspects of monkey vocalizations seem to live, too.

56

I'm not sure if we want, on the analogy to lateral language areas, to call it the "medial language area," however – medial speech area, perhaps, but these vocalizations scarcely meet our criteria for words, let alone structured language. I'm not just being picky about my terminology, however; I suspect that our kind of language didn't arise from some intensification of the usual ape vocal repertoire.

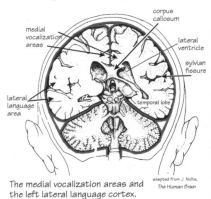

The medial vocalization areas and the left lateral language cortex.

There are several reasons to suspect this. Besides the distance (almost half the brain's width) between the two areas, there's also the meaninglessness of our phonemes, in contrast to the one-sound-one-meaning obligatory interpretation of chimpanzee vocalizations. I have trouble imagining how evolution manag-ed the trick of making some new vocalizations meaningless while retaining the obligatory meaning of the rest, during the transition period. It happened somehow, of course, but it makes me think that the meaningless additional ones didn't grow up beside the old ones in the competition for cortical space, that they got a fresh start somewhere else, perhaps not even as vocalizations. I wish we knew whether the chimps and bonobos had some intermediate specializations, especially the language-reared individuals. (Do they borrow some lateral cortex, as they come to understand all of those human sentences? Tune in next year, I'm told.)

LET ME PUT ALL OF THIS SPECIALIZED REAL ESTATE in a broader context, that of the cerebral cortex in general. It's a layered structure, mostly up on the surface of the brain abutting the skull, except for what's buried in infolding. The word "subcortical" refers to everything else in the brain. Most of our cortex is newer, mammalian-style neocortex, with six thin layers like a croissant (older parts of cortex, such as hippocampus, have only three, like cakes). And it's neocortex that has the reputation for handling novelties, such as associative memories. Subcortical structures have more of the reputation of handling subroutines, and with repetition, what is initially a cortical task may become a subcortical one. Tasks like language, full of novelty and multimodality relationships, rely heavily on the neocortex, even though coordinating performance may additionally involve structures like the thalamus and cerebellum. I'm going to stick to neocortical novelty and not attempt to make a wiring diagram of everything involved in aphasia and routine speech.

There are lots of ways to describe the real estate; motor strip (that map of the muscles at the rear of the frontal lobe) is an obvious output pathway, and there are obvious sensory input specializations such as the primary somatosensory, primary auditory, and primary visual areas. Everything else (about 85 percent of the brain's surface area) got called "association cortex."

It's not quite terra incognita, however. We started finding a number of secondary sensory maps in parts of association cortex; for vision, there are a few dozen additional maps of the visual world, some quite small.

These days, we tend to talk about the cortex's major regions as sensory and postsensory (those *what* and *where*

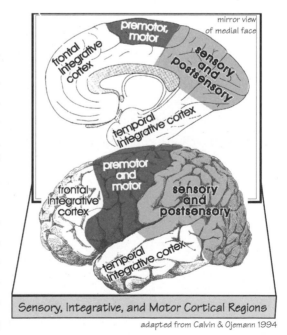

Sensory, Integrative, and Motor Cortical Regions

adapted from Calvin & Ojemann 1994

specialties occupying occipital, parietal, and some of temporal lobe), motor and premotor (in the back half of the frontal lobe), and the rest as "integrative" cortex. I still call it association cortex, myself. But notice that it has very little to do with the lobes, whose boundaries are difficult to define in any case.

There's really no "executive cortex," a spot where the big picture comes together and decisions are made. But you won't go far wrong if you think of your brain as always preparing for action, trying to guess what happens next, and gathering sensory information in aid of tentative plans for action. To the classical *who, what, where, when, why,* and *how,* there needs to be added a seventh question: *action?*

This is, you understand, a motor systems neurophysiologist speaking; others often adopt a more inside-looking-out psychological perspective. The difference in perspectives often comes to the surface when discussing consciousness; while I'm busy discussing how Darwinian processes sort through ambiguity and create novel plans of action, they usually are talking instead about awareness, how you focus your attention on various aspects of the environment.

As Gregory Bateson once said, information is data that makes a difference – that which sways your choice about what to do next. Sensory information is sometimes collected systematically or at random (we are, to some extent, "interrupt driven"). But much of the time, information from the sense organs and our memories is being collected in aid of a plan of action, one of several that are percolating up into consciousness. Each possible action triggers a number of questions, including the aforementioned *who-what-where-when-why-how.*

And that preparation for action perspective helps us to understand verbs and their needs for linking to themes–agents, beneficiaries, and so forth. As I mentioned earlier, verbs seem to live in the frontal lobe behind the temple. The most elementary verbs naturally come with arguments. A verb like "go" always needs an orientation: when *go* surfaces as an issue, secondary issues need to be decided involving where to go, toward what object or person, around what obstacles, with what means, and so forth. A verb like "give" immediately raises such issues as "give *what*" and "to *whom*," even if the giver is yourself. Because the frontal lobe is also engaged in marshaling actions over some time span (long holds, for example, are a prefrontal specialty in monkeys doing a delayed-match-to-sample task), such ancillary issues as *when* to go may be closely linked. That's why I said adverbs such as "quickly" and "slowly" likely resided in frontal lobe as well, though there's not much data yet.

And, of course, we're really talking about connotations of a word here, not its pronunciation. Sometimes a stroke patient can use a word like *crack* as a verb ("crack a nut" if they have an intact frontal lobe) but not as a noun ("a crack in a window" if they have temporal lobe damage).

NOUNS AND ADJECTIVES involve a different type of concept; they may make links but usually not obligatory ones in the demanding manner of verbs. There has been a major rearrangement of the temporal lobe that features space for concepts, one that may have something to do with the vocabulary-without-structuring stage of protolanguage. Some stroke patients can name tools, but not animals. Others are missing their plants, or body parts, or verbs, – or perhaps the combination of food, fruits, and vegetables. Mind you, they can usually *recognize* the word, and write the word. What they are usually missing is the visual representation of that category.

The secondary visual areas in the parietal and temporal lobes feature a *where-what* split, with the parietal lobe being more concerned with *where*, and the temporal lobe with the *what* issues. In monkeys, much of the temporal lobe is devoted to the *what*-type secondary visual areas; the top side of the temporal lobe is auditory. (I'm going to have to compare monkeys to humans because no one yet knows about the ape temporal lobe, though they're starting to train one of the language-reared chimpanzees in a context that allows brain scans.)

Overall, of course, the human brain is a lot bigger than monkey brains. Monkeys have about enough cerebral cortex on both sides to cover a postcard, were the thin cortical rim peeled off and flattened out. Apes (that's a bonobo at right) have enough so that it would cover a sheet of typing paper. We've got four sheets worth.

But the human cortex is rearranged, too, and temporal lobe is the best-studied case. The human temporal lobe has all of those monkey-style visual areas back in the rear, the primary auditory area on the top middle, with something else going on in the middle and front of the temporal lobe. What filled in?

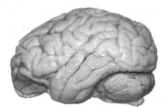

So far as neurologists can tell from studying stroke patients, the reorganized human temporal lobe is all about categories, exactly what Derek needs for protolanguage's vocabulary.

Bonobo Brain

Toward the rear are such things as color, then comes stuff more like tool concepts. The front end of the temporal lobe ("temporal tip" seems to have more to do with carefully delimited categories of one: proper nouns. Epileptic patients who have had a temporal tip surgically removed sometimes say that they're always having to write down a new name, that their recall of proper names isn't what it used to be, pre-op.

There's another way of studying concepts: try to confuse a small locality in the cortex by tingling it with a mild electrical current. The opportunities to get such data are largely come from the surgical treatment of epileptic seizures and the associated pre-op workups needed to make sure that the patient will benefit from surgery. I'll save you the details (they're in *Conversations with Neil's Brain* that George Ojemann and I wrote together) and just say that the brief stimulation doesn't evoke concepts or words, it merely prevents them from arising, despite the patient's attempt to access them. The sensitive spot for disrupting a tool concept might be no larger than a small coin (strokes usually have to be larger than that just to be noticed at all; stimulation can identify much smaller specialized regions).

THERE ARE OTHER CORTICAL LOCALES known as "naming sites" because stimulation at them causes the patient to fumble at naming any sort of common object: shown a drawing, the patient says, "This is a . . . a . . . . Oh, I know what that is, it's a . . . ." The patient can speak, but can't get out the common name; turn off the current, and the name will often pop out, finally. A half-dozen such naming sites can be found in a given patient, scattered around the temporal, parietal, and frontal lobes on the lateral surface; they're different places in different people, but usually not more than several fingers' width from the left sylvian fissure (there are probably more, buried in folds, inaccessible). Neurosurgeons are very careful to avoid these naming sites when removing epileptic tissue from the brain, for fear of creating an aphasia (a loss of language abilities). If there has to be a tradeoff, aphasia is usually considered worse than epilepsy.

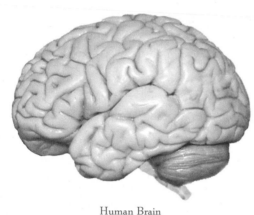

Human Brain

One fascinating aspect of naming sites is that, in bilingual patients, they are sometimes different for the different languages. Test the patient with a series of object drawings, asking him to name them in English, and find the coin-sized sites where stimulation blocks the naming ("naming sites"). Then repeat the series, asking him to name them in Spanish, or whatever. Some of the English naming sites will not block naming in Spanish; there will also be some new naming sites, where naming in Spanish is blocked but not in English. Some naming sites block both languages. The naming sites are only a small percentage of all the sites tested (imaging methods show that much wider areas of cortex are working harder during such tasks – they're *involved* but not *essential*).

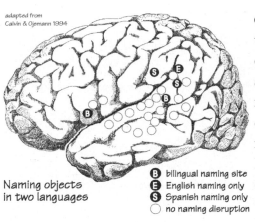

adapted from
Calvin & Ojemann 1994

Naming objects
in two languages

B bilingual naming site
E English naming only
S Spanish naming only
○ no naming disruption

The momentary electrical buzz can be used to study a number of different brain functions, a technique pioneered in middle of the twentieth century by the Montreal neurosurgeon Wilder Penfield, and greatly expanded over the last three decades by George Ojemann in Seattle. In most cases, it causes a function to fail, though in the motor cortex in the back end of the frontal lobe, it causes poorly coordinated movements. ("Hey, somebody moved my right thumb!") Crude sensory impressions can be evoked in primary sensory cortices, but usually not formed sensations. The reports of hearing music, or seeing a man walking a dog, may be related to the patient's typical aura of an impending seizure – something that the electrical buzz can provoke, if too strong. So these so-called "experiential responses" are not necessarily normal ones, but perhaps those "burned in" by previous seizures – set pieces, not easily disassociated into meaningful parts, rather like multi-word exclamations or whale songs.

WHERE, DEREK WILL SURELY ASK, are the boundary words located? Words like "since" and "because," that signal a new verb coming up? Or words like "of" and "into" that signal a new phrase? There are only a few dozen such words, a closed class that is difficult to expand (though we can always add more nouns and verbs). If the brain handled a closed-class word as a special case (in the manner of irregular verbs and nouns) in a particular place, we would have a substantial clue to how a structured sentence is parsed into smaller units.

Alas, the closed-class words have not usually been part of the experimental design for cortical localization of language, at least not thus far. Ojemann and coworkers do see cortical "grammar" sites where the patient makes mistakes when reading aloud, substituting the wrong verb endings, pronouns, conjunctions, and prepositions, but at these sites, patients don't make mistakes reading nouns and verb stems.

The loss of cortical specializations for the closed class might be important for Broca's aphasia, where language production tends to degenerate into protolanguage's short utterances. Such patients often have trouble with sentence understanding, typically with the closed-class words such as conjunctions and prepositions, even though their understanding of other word types remains.

In the Wernicke-style aphasias, understanding is often poor even though production retains phrases and clauses. Such patients talk fluently, even excessively, but they sometimes use words that make no sense. So quality isn't very good, in the manner that might be expected of a Darwinian competition that was never able to operate for enough generations before the utterance was put into action or comprehension deemed good enough.

DB: This is very striking evidence for what I think you are going to say later — that there is Darwinian competition between sentences, a process that surprisingly produces "garbage in, quality out." Because if there weren't, where would these nonsense phrases come from? What they often look like are bits of quite different sentences put together, like this one: "I'll tell I've been my wife was every time dollars for teeth and my wife didn't pay any at home."

Aphasias come in many varieties. What students, fresh from learning about sensory areas and movement areas elsewhere, tend to remember about them is a great oversimplification, but here it is: understanding depends a lot on the cortical areas bordering the rear half of the left sylvian fissure, while expression is more a matter of frontal lobe areas somewhat in front of the temporal tip. I shudder to think of all of the exceptions to this "rule."

During the first century of neurology, the aphasias provided an insight into cerebral localization of function for language via their correlation with surgical and postmortem findings. But the aphasia subcategories which were invented then have not, so far, meshed well with those from the more modern physiological techniques. One reason is that the cortical stimulation technique revealed that the areas surrounding the sylvian fissure specialize in both sensation and movement, at least when novel sequences are involved.

The experimental design for stimulation mapping tried, for this case, to avoid issues of language understanding by using sound sequences and movement sequences that were linguistically meaningless. For example, the patient sees a cartoon sequence of three frames, with one of the experimenters modeling three oral-facial postures: puff out cheeks, stick out tongue, clench the teeth. And so the well-trained patient does all three actions, in that order. Another cartoon slide comes up, and the patient does another three. Stimulation occurs during some slides, but not during others; it's so weak that he doesn't know when it is occurring. During stimulation, he may produce the movements, but in the wrong order. Or he may add movements not modeled on the current slide. If the cartoon series is simply the same posture repeated three times, the patient makes no errors. Stimulation is only disrupting when a sequence of *different* movements must be produced.

Movements are supposed to be a frontal lobe function, but movement sequencing seems to involve the temporal and the parietal lobe as well, at some sites near the sylvian fissure. At about 86 percent of these movement-sequencing sites, a listening-to-sound-sequences task is similarly disrupted, so it looks as if this region near the sylvian fissure, front and back, has a major role in both incoming and outgoing *sequences*. This had been suspected from aphasic patients, because so many of them suffered from an inability to perform hand-arm maneuvers of a novel kind. So add hand-arm to oral-facial, and you have the picture of a common-core facility. If anything is at its center, it's probably primary auditory cortex (located on the top of the temporal lobe, largely buried in the sylvian fissure, about halfway along its length)–and certainly *not* that primate exclamation area halfway across the brain above the corpus callosum.

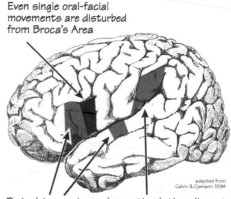

Even single oral-facial movements are disturbed from Broca's Area

adapted from Calvin & Ojemann 1994

Perisylvian regions where stimulation disrupts both phoneme receptive sequences and oral-facial expression sequences

In a rim around the perisylvian sequencing core, there are a number of sites in the frontal, parietal and temporal lobes where stimulation disrupts short-term memory tasks. But first I'd better explain some of the current concepts of how memory works in the brain, because it isn't much like the way it works in a computer.

6

How Are Memories Stored?

Computers have three levels of memory, as I was breathlessly explaining this morning on the pre-breakfast hike around Bellagio (hiking uphill enforces brevity – every writer should try this as a warmup). First, there is the type-ahead keyboard buffer, that stores your keystrokes if you're a faster typist than I am.

Eventually the letters are fetched and moved into RAM, the fast-access temporary memory that the programs utilize. It has one disadvantage (besides cost), which is the fact that everything in it is lost when the power is turned off. It's sometimes called volatile memory because the data "evaporates."

From RAM, you can move the string of letters to the hard disk, where they survive even if the power fails. All three types of computer memory have the bad habit of filling up, mostly because they use pigeonholes, a physical slot for each item of information, each with its own

> We hear and apprehend only what we already half know.
> HENRY DAVID THOREAU

address that provides the means of finding what's been stored.

Superficially, human memory looks as if it has similar functional subdivisions. There's an immediate memory, a sensory buffer (cells tend to fire for a short while, even after a sensory stimulus is over). There is a volatile short-term memory. This is sometimes called "working memory," as it's what you need to hang onto a phone number long enough to dial it; it's also what you need to repeat back a sentence, as when swearing an oath. It involves lingering traces that assist in recreating the firing patterns anytime in the next few minutes.

Finally there is a process (called "consolidation" and requiring days to accomplish) by which some short-term memory items are made into more durable long-term memories, ones that can survive the disruptive events (concussions, coma, seizures) that would fog or erase short-term memories that hadn't been consolidated yet.

But long-term memory doesn't fill up, nor does it seem to have an addressing scheme that we can discover, probably because it doesn't use pigeonholes. When you learn someone's name for the first time, you don't store it in an empty slot, as in a hard disk. You appear to store it redundantly in a number of places, overlapping it with all the previous memories stored in those places. It's a distributed memory system. Think of the storage method as being like your favorite washboarded road, the one that tries to shake your car apart at a certain speed – but one that also has resonances for trucks overlain on the washboarding that affects cars.

IN THE FIRST HALF OF THE TWENTIETH CENTURY, such facts about memory were established and, in 1949, Donald Hebb created our modern formulation of the relation between short- and long-term memories.

Impressed by the fragile nature of short-term memories, and the length of the consolidation period before some became more permanent long-term memories, he said that concepts were implemented by a characteristic firing pattern in a small group of cortical neurons, which he dubbed a cell-assembly. To recall someone's name, you needed to recreate that musical spatiotemporal firing pattern. But, because of the way that a long-term memory survived episodes such as coma and seizures, it had to be a spatial-only pattern like those washboarding ruts, something that didn't require ongoing neural activity such as impulses firing away.

It's all very much like the dominant technological metaphor of Hebb's time, the phonograph. The long-lasting grooves in the record, when a needle was dragged through them, served to recreate a spatiotemporal pattern called music or speech. And the spatial-only patterns in the grooves had been created by a spatiotemporal pattern during recording, the same one (within limits) as was later recreated.

The brain's storage method is not two-dimensional, like the record groove. Three dimensions are available, and so is redundancy (as we currently see for computer communications protocols, such as error-correcting codes). On the other hand, there are potential confusions, such as "recording over" previous material – and yet we somehow retrieve the desired item amidst the mix. A modern formulation tends to use terms such as "chaotic attractor" rather than resonance, helping to emphasize the way variant patterns are conformed to a standard. I tend, following the lead of Hebb's contemporary J. W. S. Pringle, to emphasize the role of a plainchant chorus, utilizing those redundant "grooves," helping to produce a standard version from all the potential variability caused by overwritings.

Confusing things further is that different areas of the brain are important for short-term memory than for long-term memory. It's pretty clear that neocortical areas are where most of the language-accessible long-term memories are kept, but they'll never be consolidated there unless the hippocampus is functioning well during the short-term memory period following input. People with damage to the hippocampus (and adjacent cortical areas in the midline face of the temporal lobes, common in Alzheimer's dementia) may be able to retrieve old long-term memories but they aren't forming new ones very well because consolidation doesn't work right. Yesterday may be lost to them, even though their youth is not.

This is a problem totally unlike the "emeritus professor problem" of knowing so much that it takes a long time to sort through it, and thus complaining about "memory problems." Emeritus professors (actually, the problems start in the forties for many people, professorial or not) nearly always come up with the right name eventually, proving that it was there all along. This suggests the problem is simply one of lengthening access times, where you cannot keep up with the windows of opportunity afforded by social repartee.

Brain imaging techniques utilizing regional blood flow changes are capable of seeing what areas are working harder during certain memory tasks. When a subject is given a working memory task, one analogous to the telephone operator giving you a new number that you have to remember long enough to dial, the frontal lobe areas just in front of the motor strip seem to work harder, as do the areas in the back end of the sylvian fissure. Both Broca's area and Wernicke's area, in the old formulation of language areas, are involved in working memory of this type.

Stimulation mapping of the exposed cortical surface of epileptic patients undergoing neurosurgery reveals an even more detailed picture of short-term memory. The patient watches a series of slides, a new one popping up every six

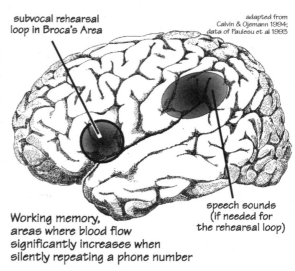

subvocal rehearsal loop in Broca's Area

adapted from Calvin & Ojemann 1994; data of Paulesu et al 1993

speech sounds (if needed for the rehearsal loop)

Working memory, areas where blood flow significantly increases when silently repeating a phone number

seconds. The first one reads, "This is a" and then shows a drawing of a common object. So the patient says, "This is an apple." The second slide will be a distraction of some sort, such as showing a two-digit number from which the patient counts backwards by threes. Then the third slide comes up, merely saying, "RECALL." The patient is supposed to say, "Apple" (or whatever the earlier object was). During some of the slides, stimulation occurs as the neurosurgeon moves around, testing different cortical sites, checking accuracy of retrieval. Stimulation of some sites in the temporal lobe during the first or second slide causes errors during recall

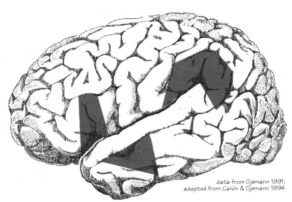

data from Ojemann 1991;
adapted from Calvin & Ojemann 1994

Zones (arbitrary) where stimulation disrupts short-term post-distractional memory

attempts (a period when there isn't stimulation), even when they didn't interfere with naming or with the distraction task. Frontal lobe stimulation sites have effects mostly when applied during the retrieval attempt itself.

The effective sites are collectively known as "short-term post-distractional memory sites" because of the suggestion that in this test, the first slide's name was either stored there or that the site had important connections to the retrieval process, allowing the electrical buzz to interfere with the recall attempt. These sites were usually located somewhat outside the perisylvian core of sequencing sites, forming something of a periphery around it. The sites affecting reading ("grammar sites") were often in between the sequencing core and the memory periphery.

There is a great deal of individual variation in the brain's language organization, some of it correlated with verbal IQ. Most dramatically, language mapping varies by sex, the male brain having many more naming sites at the back end of the sylvian fissure, the female more naming sites in the frontal lobe. The female arrangement seems more resistant to aphasia by strokes; four out of five aphasics are men. Even with the same amount of cortical damage from the stroke, the woman has much less functional impairment. As age-related mortality has long suggested, the female body plan seems to be the more secure one, less liable to serious trouble.

NONE OF THIS EXPLAINS HOW THE NEURONS accomplish these functions – or how they differ in different areas – but I hope that the foregoing explains why brain researchers expect to find the mind in the brain. I attempted a short course on cortical neurons and their synapses in the sixth chapter of *Conversations with Neil's Brain*. Then, in the first few chapters of *The Cerebral Code*, I addressed spatiotemporal patterning much more explicitly and geared up to tackle the problem of a Darwinian process (anything that mimics the full-scale copying competition that bootstraps quality, I call a "Darwin Machine"). A Darwin Machine in the cerebral cortex might operate on the time scale of thought and action, exactly what language needs. Much of the two chapters that follow are my attempt to briefly describe the basic principles and how they apply to convergent and divergent thinking.

Back in 1996, as I finished correcting the page proof of *Cerebral Code*, I realized that the long-distance common code problem (the spatiotemporal firing pattern characterizing a phrase such as "The cat on the mat" temporarily needs to be the same in the temporal lobe as it is in the frontal lobe), which I had found a technical solution for, also provided a powerful mechanism to facilitate the nested embedding of structured language. At the last minute, I added a few extra pages commenting on the subject in the final chapter of *Code*, but here I can be much more explicit about embedding and on-the-fly associations (though at the expense of being rather too brief on the underlying cellular neurophysiology). Together with the related Darwinian process that helps shape new ideas in the brain, it gives a glimpse of how higher intellectual functions might arise from lowly cells and circuits.

7

Hexagonal Mosaics
and Darwin Machines

Brains contain almost 100 billion (10^{11}) neurons in the cerebral cortex alone, and some other parts of the brain have many more neurons. Pyramidal neurons, which are tall neurons with triangular-shaped cell bodies, are the most numerous of the cortical neurons. They have a splendid dendritic tree, ascending a millimeter or two toward the cortical surface and breaking into a number of finer branches, seeking out inputs.

For output, they have a single axon leaving the cell body; it is thinner than the finest spider thread. After going a ways, the axon starts to branch as well, finally breaking into many thousands of terminal branches. Some of the branches terminate in a synapse only 0.1 mm away; others may terminate 1,000 mm away in the spinal cord. Because the synapse mostly works in only one direction, each axon branch is effectively a one-way street – all in the same direction, away from the tall tree of the dendrites and toward the axon endings. Simple back-and-forth circuits nearly

In any case, contemplating the form of the cells was one of my most beloved pleasures. Because even from an aesthetic point of view the nervous tissue has fascinating beauty. Are there in our parks any more elegant and lush trees than the Purkinje neuron in the cerebellum or the so-called psychical cell, that is, the famous cortical pyramidal neuron?

SANTIAGO RAMÓN Y CAJAL, 1923

76

always involve several neurons, just as one-way streets tend to come in pairs.

A synapse is a little gap between two adjacent cells, a border-crossing point where perfumelike neurotransmitter molecules are wafted into the no man's land and signal the specialized sniffers on the dendrite of the downstream cell (that's why synapses are mostly one-way: only one side releases packets of the neurotransmitter molecules) that something is happening up-stream. Release of neurotransmitter happens when a brief electrical impulse (also known as a spike or action potential) is

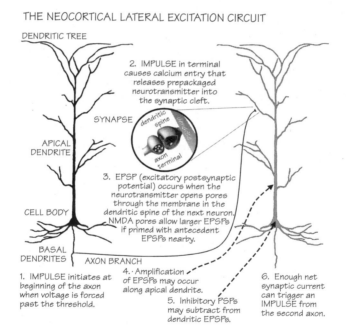

THE NEOCORTICAL LATERAL EXCITATION CIRCUIT

DENDRITIC TREE

2. IMPULSE in terminal causes calcium entry that releases prepackaged neurotransmitter into the synaptic cleft.

SYNAPSE

dendritic spine

axon terminal

APICAL DENDRITE

3. EPSP (excitatory postsynaptic potential) occurs when the neurotransmitter opens pores through the membrane in the dendritic spine of the next neuron. NMDA pores allow larger EPSPs if primed with antecedent EPSPs nearby.

CELL BODY

BASAL DENDRITES

AXON BRANCH

1. IMPULSE initiates at beginning of the axon when voltage is forced past the threshold.

4. Amplification of EPSPs may occur along apical dendrite.

5. Inhibitory PSPs may subtract from dendritic EPSPs.

6. Enough net synaptic current can trigger an IMPULSE from the second axon.

sent from the beginning of the axon near the cell body. It propagates down the axon and out all its fine branches, releasing packets of the neurotransmitter chemical (in these pyramidal neurons, the amino acid called "glutamate") from the axon terminals when the impulse finally reaches them.

On the other side of the synapse, the neurotransmitter causes (via that sniffer mechanism) a small voltage change in the downstream neuron known as an excitatory postsynaptic potential (EPSP). A number of such inputs are usually required to trigger an impulse in the downstream neuron; this threshold for impulse production means that the neurons even further downstream aren't told anything about what's happening upstream unless a sufficient number of the right types of inputs have coordinated their actions. A chain of neurons represents a cascade of thresholds to be overcome, so most chains are silent much of the time.

The other major type of cortical neuron is called stellate; it lacks the tall dendrite, having only bushy ones, and therefore looks more like a shrub than a tree. It works just like the others except for releasing a different neurotransmitter chemical, typically called GABA. This different scent wafted across the synaptic no-mans-land has an inhibitory action on its downstream neurons, a negative voltage change (the IPSP) that reduces any positive EPSPs.

The dendrites of a pyramidal neuron receive about 10,000 inputs; 8,000 synapses are excitatory, and 2,000 inhibitory. Their actions add and subtract like deposits and withdrawals from a bank account – though sometimes with nonlinear double-your-money features rarely provided by banks. But most synapses are silent at any given moment, with only a few hundred needed to put the neuron through its paces, ranging from barely firing to repeatedly firing as fast as possible. In general, you can think of the pyramidal neurons as the excitatory ones, and the stellates as the inhibitory ones.

To summarize this simplified cellular neurophysiology, voltage changes are the basis of computation (you add and subtract with PSPs, trying to exceed a voltage threshold). Voltage change is also the basis of the communication of the computational result (impulses propagate over long distances, then release neurotransmitter). The synapses are just, so far, a primitive way of passing voltage changes across the gap between adjacent cells, something like changing Italian lira for Swiss francs when crossing the border west of Lake Como.

But synapses are also the most easily altered link in this chain of intracellular events, the major way of adjusting the strength of the excitatory or inhibitory influence, of making an input twice as influential as it was before. Synapses are the volume controls of the brain, what affects how "loudly" one neuron "hears" another. The arriving impulse can release more packets of neurotransmitter than before. Previously ineffective postsynaptic channels can also be brought on line, augmenting the effect of a standard dose of neurotransmitter via having more sniffers.

This altered strength is usually temporary, fading in seconds or minutes, but it can be made relatively permanent during consolidation. In combination with many other synapses in an ensemble of neurons, it is what records new memories. More indiscriminate changes in synaptic strength, affecting many cells at once, are how most mind-altering chemicals work, such as stimulants and anesthetics, as well as the major psychiatric medications.

CIRCUITS INVOLVING A NUMBER OF NEURONS can do things that a single neuron cannot. They can create precision timing between impulses, free of jitter in a way that no one lonely unconnected neuron could ever manage to do. They can also create complex patterns between neurons: eighty-eight neurons, each hooked up to a piano key, could play little tunes of some complexity. When I use the term "spatiotemporal pattern," just think of an ensemble of neurons (sometimes more than 88) creating a distinctive little pattern of firing, rather like a line of melody.

Just as any one pixel of a computer screen participates at various times in many different patterns representing different letters and drawings, so any one neuron participates in many committees. Each committee generates a different tune. Though we tend to focus on the neuron as the unit of computation and the synapse as a site of modifiability, the pattern's the thing, much as it is on a computer screen. To understand how concepts, words, phrases, clauses, and sentences are represented – and how they compete with one another, to shape up quality – we have to understand the elementary patterns on which other patterns build.

Shortly, I'm going to claim that one little tune is the code *A* for apple and that other tunes (more like symphonies with a number of different voices) create a temporary code for a sentence. Each of those tunes can play from a "keyboard" about 300 notes long, whose neurons are contained in a cortical space about 0.5 mm across, shaped like a hexagon. The tuneful hexagons always exist redundantly in a little hexagonal mosaic of identical clones, like that synchronized chorus I mentioned when introducing Pringle's 1951 insight. I hope that this will serve as motivation to learn the cortical circuitry that serves as the basis for the hexagons that ought to emerge now and then in the electrical activity.

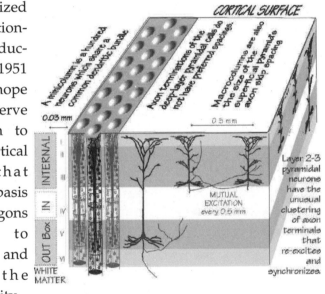

SYNCHRONIZATION OF CORTICAL NEURONS can occur via a number of mechanisms, but the one of most interest for our present purposes involves a peculiar property of the axon of a pyramidal neuron in the upper layers of neocortex. The axon acts like an express train, skipping many intermediate stops, giving off synapses only when about 0.5, 1.0, and 1.5 mm away from the tall dendrite (and sometimes continuing for a few millimeters farther, maintaining the integer multiples of the basic metric, 0.5 mm). These express axons spread sideways in the cortex, remaining within the superficial layers and synapsing mostly with other pyramidal neurons in the superficial layers of 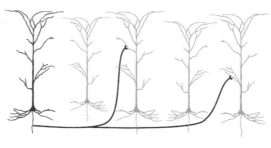 neocortex. The same originating pyramidal neuron has, of course, other axon branches (it has nearly 10,000 total) that burrow into the white matter and travel long distances front and back, left and right, but the express train arrangement is a property of their axons that stay near home, not straying very far from their layers of origin. The pyramidal neurons of the deeper cortical layers also have recurrent excitation, but their sideways axon branches don't seem to have the express train gaps where synapses are omitted (they're the "all-stops" trains).

Neuroanatomists have seen variants on the superficial layer express train patterning in most cortical areas, and in most mammals, that they have examined thus far. I have predicted – in *The Cerebral Code* – what some of the physiological consequences might be, and when our physiological recording and imaging techniques improve in resolution, we can begin to answer such important questions as how often and where the predicted Darwinian processes occur. For the moment, what follows has the status of a theoretical prediction based on neuroanatomy, not physiological data.

Because neurons of a particular cortical area all have about the same gap length, there's a good chance of two neurons talking to one another; that is, reciprocally exciting one another. While this might produce the circuitry needed for an impulse to chase its tail, round and round between neurons, I doubt that this is a common occurrence. The most likely consequence of this mutual connectivity is that the two neurons will often fire at about the same time. Many models of coupled oscillators exhibit such entrainment; it was first reported in 1665 by the Danish physicist Christian Huygens, who noticed that two pendulum clocks sitting on the same shelf would synchronize their ticks via vibrations within a half hour after being started at different times. Fireflies do the same thing much more quickly; whole trees full of fireflies can be observed, flashing in synchrony.

The express train anatomy in the superficial layers of cortex suggests that neurons 0.5 mm apart in triangular arrays might be firing in synchrony on many occasions, even when in-between neurons are not. As the background balance of excitation and inhibition varies, you'd expect to see a given triangular array extend its reach for many millimeters, then contract into just a few nodes, then disappear entirely. These patterns are ephemeral.

Furthermore, there might be another triangular array, 0.2 mm away from the first, firing in synchrony but at a different time than the first triangular array. Indeed, there could be hundreds of triangular arrays, each firing at different times, but I doubt if that happens very often; a dozen seems quite sufficient, just as you'd seldom use more than a dozen keys on a piano for a simple tune, even though 88 are available. Just think of a roomful of player pianos, all playing the same tune in lockstep.

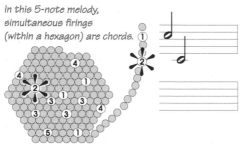

In this 5-note melody, simultaneous firings (within a hexagon) are chords.

So how many keys does the cortical piano have? Well, the largest collection of active nodes (from all arrays taken together) that has no redundancies (just one member of each active array) could be no larger than a hexagon 0.5 mm across (the corresponding points − say the upper left corners – of a mosaic of hexagonal tiles are always connected by triangular arrays). Within a 0.5 mm hexagon of neocortex are about 30,000 neurons, but they often function together in units of about 100 neurons, each called a minicolumn (the orientation columns of visual cortex are the most familiar example, where all neurons seem to be interested in the same thing, lines and edges tilted at the same angle to the visual vertical). Because there are about 300 units within a hexagon, think of a piano keyboard 300 keys long, each key mapped to a particular minicolumn and sounding whenever a cell in that minicolumn fires. And think of not just one megapiano but a whole chorus of them, expanding to recruit more megapianos nearby.

Once two hexagons get their little tune going (and, you realize, that spatiotemporal pattern is what I was referring to, when I talked of the code *A* that represented *apple*), they can recruit neighboring hexagons; this probably happens one triangular array at a time but, when they've all recruited new nodes in an adjacent space, it's as if a hexagon had been cloned.

It's like a plainchant choir, recruiting additional singers. But it's all very ephemeral, here one second and gone the next. Yet I consider it the basis of working memory, and an excellent candidate for how a Darwinian process could function in the brain to improve quality. Indeed, I discovered it because I was on the lookout for cortical circuitry that could support Darwin's recursive bootstrapping of quality, on the time scale of thought and action.

DARWIN'S DISCOVERY ABOUT HOW EVOLUTION could occur in a simple, almost automatic way revolutionized our notions about how complex plants and animals came into being. Though often summarized by Darwin's phrase, "natural selection," it's really a process with six essential ingredients; when any are missing, interesting things may still happen but the recursive aspect is missing, what allows the course to be repeated for additional credit. The cortical entrainment circuitry is how you get started with a Darwinian process in the cortex, operating on the time scale of thought and action, shaping up perceptions, ideas, and action plans into higher and higher quality.

A good cloning mechanism is not, of course, the whole Darwinian quality improvement process. So far as I can tell, you need

(1) a characteristic pattern (like that A melody) that can

(2) be copied, with

(3) occasional variations (A') or compounding, where

(4) populations of A and A' compete for a limited territory, their relative success biased by

(5) a multifaceted environment (Darwin's *natural selection*), and where

(6) the next round of variants is primarily based on the more successful of the current generation (Darwin's *inheritance principle*).

There are some other things, such as sex and environmental fluctuations, which will make the Darwinian process operate faster, but they're optional – you can get the recursive boot-strapping of quality without them. A lot of things loosely called "Darwinian" may involve only some of the essentials – say, neural development where a pattern is created by selective removal of connections biased by a multifaceted environment. They're interesting and very useful, but they exhibit no copying, have no populations to compete, and lack a next generation biased by antecedent success. They're not able to repeat the course for additional credit – as you can do with a full-fledged Darwinian process. Such recursion is how you bootstrap quality, why we can start with subconscious thoughts as jumbled as our night time dreams and still end up with a sentence of quality or a logical expression. You need a quality bootstrapping mechanism in order to figure out what to do with leftovers in the refrigerator; with successive attempts running through your head as you stand there with the door open, you can often find a "quality" scheme, that is, one that doesn't require another trip to the grocery store.

The focus on what sort of ensemble activity could be cloned (#2) actually serves to define the unit pattern (#1), the spatiotemporal firing pattern in a few hundred minicolumns within a 0.5 mm hexagon. (That is, by the way, how the DNA sequence pattern was discovered to be the genetic message: Crick and Watson were searching for what molecule could be reliably copied during mitosis.) To get variants, cloning needs to be slightly imperfect – and that's not difficult when hexagonal mosaics are still small. Just as thick fingers might strike two piano keys at once or land on a neighboring key, so variants in the spatiotemporal pattern (#3) can easily arise, particularly when inexcitable hexagons limit the number of neighboring hexagons to only two or three. If the variant "breeds true" by cloning, then one can have two different populations that can compete with each other (#4), rather as bluegrass and crabgrass compete for my back yard.

One pattern may do better than the other because of the cortex's multifaceted environment. Just as bluegrass may do better than crabgrass because of your attempts to cut it regularly, water it, fertilize it, and so forth, so cortex has a number of factors that together allow one pattern to clone territory better than its competitors (#5). They include current sensory inputs to the cortex beneath the competing patterns, the background of neuromodulators (the mix of serotonin, dopamine, norepi-nephrine, acetylcholine, and a flock of peptides), and the "washboarded road" of the synaptic strengths that allow some patterns to resonate well – in other words, memories.

Finally, we need a cortical version of Darwin's inheritance principle (#6), which will preferentially create the next generation of variants from the more numerous of the current patterns. This happens because large hexagonal mosaics have more perimeter than the smaller, less successful ones – and the periphery is the only place that pattern copying can escape perfect cloning, where they have fewer than six identical neighbors to conform them to the standardized pattern. The mosaic's periphery is also where the variant A' has an unpatterned territory next door, available for colonization. There A' can "set up shop" and go into competition with its parent pattern A. So a more successful pattern has a larger territory –

which has more edge length, and therefore more opportunities to generate new variants – than do the less successful of the patterns.

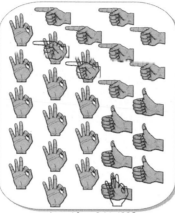

Deciding to act might be a matter of cloning movement commands. Movement might not be initiated until one dominates.

A competition for cortical territory might occur as overlapping patterns are converted into one or the other, depending in part on fading resonances from earlier occupations.

adapted from Calvin 1996

If the background level of neuromodulators or neurotransmitters fades, a large hexagonal mosaic will be broken up into a series of small mosaics, with abandoned territories in between where triangular arrays could not be maintained. This population crash is what happens to animal populations during a drought; it's also like what happens when rising sea level fragments a low-land population into subpopulations on a series of hilltops, now called islands. All of the sudden, there is a lot more perimeter, many more chances for new variants to get started.

Environmental fluctuations and islands may not be essential for a Darwinian process to recursively bootstrap quality, but they can certainly speed up the process. Judging from the "waves" of the EEG, the cortex has lots of excitability fluctuations that cover a few square centimeters of cortex, able to pump up quality via a series of population crashes and re-expansions. If a Darwinian process is to operate quickly enough to produce good results within the behavioral windows of opportunity, it may need all the known catalysts.

SYSTEMATIC RECOMBINATION is the other major catalyst. We tend to think of variants as arising from mutations, but evolution wouldn't have gotten very complex without some more systematic ways of making errors and encouraging new combinations. Bacterial conjugation serves to mix up the genes of several individuals; sex is a more systematic way of doing the same thing.

In cortex, variants may arise at the periphery but there are several ways to perform superpositions of two patterns. The first naturally arises when two different hexagonal mosaics meet: they may override, if sufficiently different; the musical analogy would be two-part singing, just as in the medieval elaboration of plainchant into several voices. Some patterns go together better than others; the same melody displaced up a fifth or an octave works well, and the later development of major and minor scales provide other examples.

Going together well in cortex ("harmony") is probably a matter of the multifaceted environment; copying mechanisms could temporarily maintain any two overlapped patterns, but only those combination patterns that resonate well with the "washboarded road" of synaptic strengths and current sensory inputs might be able to continue, once imposed copying faded next door and the spatiotemporal firing pattern had to sustain itself like a choir without prompts from the choirmaster.

WHILE THE REAL STRENGTH of a Darwinian process is for divergent thinking (creativity, where there is no right answer), it can also be used for convergent thinking when the answer isn't obvious. Sometimes you have to guess well, as when acoustics or conflicting overheard conversations force you to guess the words that you missed hearing (a substantial problem at the Villa Serbelloni when the dining room is full and dozens of voices are bouncing off the stone walls). So let me use the word-guessing problem as an example of how a Darwinian process can help you make a good (though not necessarily correct) guess.

DB: It's been reckoned, I'm not sure quite how, that languages are about 50 percent redundant, that is, you could hear only 50 percent of the acoustic signal – provided it's in your native language – and still understand everything that was intended. Under poor conditions, at cocktail parties or rock concerts, you may lose 50 percent and have to ask people to repeat. Under moderate conditions, you won't even notice a missing 20 or 30 percent.

Several things help if we hear "b-or-p, l, *unidentified vowel*, ck." One is acoustic space around words. I mean, the following are all possible English words: black, bleck, blick, block, bluck, plack, pleck, plick, plock, pluck, blag, bleg, blig, blog, blug, plag, pleg, plig, plog, plug. But out of those twenty very similar sounding words, only four are actually kosher English words (plus "blag," which is British criminal slang for robbery with violence), which means if we only partially hear a word, we have many fewer possibilities to sort through.

Whew! So let's assume that you heard Derek's ambiguous sound string, "b-or-p, l, *unidentified vowel*, ck" in the context of, say, "a big _____ dog," and you need to develop some candidates for what it might be. The first candidate you encounter may be so good, so "right" by pragmatic criteria, that no Darwinian competition is necessary. But let's assume it is harder, that you need a runoff once you develop a few candidates.

The received sound string will constitute a little tune, once encoded into ensemble firing patterns (which, of course, are quite abstract compared to the sound features, rather like hash codes). Imagine a whole hexagonal mosaic of X, what we'll call the sensory buffer, abutting a fallow field – a field full of resonances with common words, but with no cloned spatiotemporal patterning at the moment. The first problem is to produce some variant patterns, X', X'', X''', and so forth. That's most easily

88

done with a series of barriers, each with a slit that temporarily reduces the number of possible neighbors capable of correcting an error in copying. The barrier is simply a string of hexagons with insufficient excitation to support recruitment by expansionistic triangular arrays. The slit is more than two, and less than three, hexagons wide (a bit more than a millimeter); the pair of hexagons in the slit are as excitable as those in the sensory buffer that cloned them. But as they go to clone a vacant hexagon in the fallow

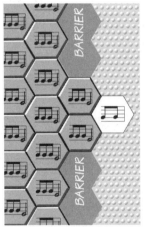

A BARRIER will not support triangular array extension. The reasons might be anatomical (lack of standard-length axon segments) or temporary (insufficient background excitation).

A GATEWAY is an excitable gap in the barrier, about two hexagons wide, where the loss of error correcting neighbors can permit variants to arise.
Adapted from Calvin 1996

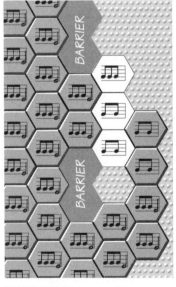

THE END RUN. If two copies of the same variant get started, this novel spatiotemporal pattern may be able to clone. If it is closer to a basin of attraction, it may successfully compete for territory with the parent pattern.

cortex to the right, they may make a mistake, perhaps omitting one of the hexagon's triangular arrays, perhaps committing the thick finger error of hitting upon the wrong minicolumn. Should this error happen in the first two hexagons filled, to the right of the slit, the modified pattern X' may take off, cloning its own territory and conforming all the surrounded hexagons with the new standard pattern X'. When X' passes through another slit, we get more errors that clone themselves, resulting in X'', and so forth. So you get variations on a theme, much as in Derek's example: black, bleck, blick, block, bluck, plack, pleck, plick, plock, pluck, plug.

But only four variations are likely to find resonances, the ones that have been heard so often in the past that they formed resonances in the synaptic strength patterns underlying the fallow field. And so, only black, block, plug, and pluck are likely to maintain hexagonal territories, once the sensory buffer stops driving the action in the formerly fallow field. We have found some candidates for the ambiguous sound string; now we have to make a decision via a Darwinian copying competition.

DB: Context will help here – if we hear "b-or-p, l, *unidentified vowel*, ck" in the context "a big _____ dog," then we know it's not likely to be "a pluck dog" or "a block dog," it's most probably "a black dog."

Context can eliminate a lot of possibilities, and our heads are full of second-order associations like "red robin," which also appear as resonances (perhaps elsewhere, rather than in the same formerly fallow field; I'll tell you in a minute how we can transfer this competition to a new playing field in some distant area of the brain). Pretty soon, the hexagons that code for "black" have cloned a lot more territory than the others, simply because there weren't many resonances for the combinations of "pluck dog" and "block dog." The blacks don't have to wipe out the competition, merely attain enough of a plurality to function in another competition, the one that will be concerned with the meaning of an entire noun phrase. All this presumably happens (we don't actually know yet) in the half-second or so that it takes to analyze and respond to such pattern recognition tasks. If everything had to be done by trying first one thing and then another, it would probably take minutes, but the brain likely has a lot of neural machinery operating in parallel on the problem.

DB: Another thing is all those articles and prepositions, those near meaningless bits of words that make up so surprisingly much of our speech – these all serve as signposts, so to speak, to the syntactic structure. The structure tells you what class a misheard word probably belongs to, and this in turn reduces the possibilities to very few or often just one.

Variants can also be creative, especially the ones for combination codes; by mixing up features of a horse and a rhinoceros, you can create never-seen creatures such as a unicorn. Indeed, it is the usefulness of the Darwinian process for divergent thinking that is its most intriguing application, with the promise of explaining much of our subconscious evolution of thoughts and how they might be shaped into collections of higher quality than the jumbled juxtapositions of our nighttime dreams. I assume that the sentences we eventually speak start out as low-quality collections, not making good sense – and even when they do, that they need a lot of improvement to put them in a form so that others might understand them. As speakers, we have to find the right word choices and arrangements that help the listener to quickly guess our who-did-what-to-whom mental model.

I'll address the issue of how we speak a sentence we've never spoken before, but after another short dose of cortical neuro-physiology: tackling the long-distance issues, important for how we tie together the multimodality aspects of a concept.

THE CONCEPT SITES THAT WE SAW IN THE PREVIOUS CHAPTERS could just be areas with the right resonances. They need not, in this two-level Hebbian view, actually be pure specialists; they need only be sites for the right long-term resonances, with the ephemeral spatiotemporal firing patterns there often representing something else, such as the X'' variants of the Darwinian workspace.

I said that resonances often exhibited "capture" effects: let any active pattern come close to the resonance, and it will be forced into the memorized resonance (just think of how the washboarded road forces you to slow down, making the jarring even more prominent). While there can be temporary spatiotemporal patterns that represent the unknowns of the sensory world, the resonances mean that some hexagonal firing patterns like A represent familiar features of a former environment, such as an apple. It's the widespread repetitions of the resonance that constitute the distributed nature of the memory; you can resurrect the active firing pattern A from any of a number of pairs of hexagons in the utilized regions of cerebral cortex.

Now the problem is: How do you communicate this code to a distant patch of cortex? And the answer to that will also show how on-the-fly trial associations can be done, such as that "block dog" and "black dog."

8

A Common Code:
The Brain's "Esperanto" Problem

Many of our concepts have multiple sensory modalities associated with them. The flowers in the formal gardens that cascade below the Villa Serbelloni have, in my head, both a visual category and an associated smell (and often an associated insect!), from all my trips up the path.

If the concept is a word, it also has some associated movements, needed to pronounce or write the word. Neocortex is where the sight of a comb, say, is matched up to the feel of a comb in your hand. While the spatiotemporal firing patterns for the comb's sight and feel are likely different, they become to be associated in the cortex – along with those for hearing the sound /k m/ or hearing the characteristic sounds that the teeth of a comb make when they're plucked. Any of these inputs could enable you to say, "That's a *comb*." On the production side, you not only have linked spatiotemporal patterns for pronouncing /k m/ but also ones for manipulating a comb through the hair on your head, or for writing down the word on your list of left-behind items that need to be replaced on a walk down into the streets of Bellagio. There are likely a dozen different cortical codes associated with combs, all located (as Sigmund Freud suspected a century ago) in different places in the cortex. How can we link them? Say, link the concepts of the temporal lobe with the verbs of the frontal lobe?

The largest bundle of nerve fibers in the brain is the corpus callosum – which, as every intro psych student knows, connects the right brain with the left brain. But the second largest is the arcuate fasciculus, connecting the temporal lobe with the frontal lobe on the same side. The left arcuate fasciculus has got to be heavily involved in communicating temporal lobe concepts to any sentence-planning machinery in the frontal lobe part of the language system. There are subcortical paths involving chains of neurons in the thalamus or basal ganglia that also connect the two lobes, but the arcuate fasciculus is largely made up of the direct corticocortical paths; they're branches of the same sideways axons whose express train patterning created all the interesting possibilities for cloning spatiotemporal patterns.

The arcuate fasciculus is a mere pipeline, analogous to a fiber optic bundle of thousands of thin light pipes. It is not like the better kinds of fiber optic bundles, the coherent type that they use for endoscopes. When neighboring fibers at one end aren't still neighbors by the time they reach the far end, having gotten jumbled somewhere along the way, such bundles are called "incoherent." Used for viewing some internal organ, displacements would occur, rather like the way Picasso put eyes in the middle of foreheads. Even when nothing as dramatic as jumble happens in our cerebral pathways, things are still blurred because each fiber fans out at the far end, spanning a millimeter or more.

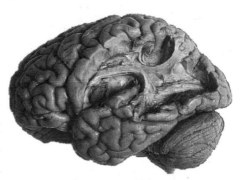

What all this incoherence means is that the firing pattern within a neural committee (what Hebb called a cell-assembly, and what I claim can be contained in a

Frontal- to temporal-lobe pathway
(arcuate fasciculus)

half-millimeter hexagonal patch of cortex) cannot be communicated undistorted to another region of the brain – not the way it could if the arcuate fasciculus were as coherent as the fiber optics in an endoscope. I'm not going to propose that the overall size of the arcuate fasciculus has changed disproportionately, only that the "choirs" that drive it on occasion finally become large enough to achieve coherent transmission, perhaps because the Darwinian competition in the sending cortex grew a particularly extensive hexagonal mosaic.

FORTUNATELY, THE JUMBLE AND BLUR aren't really a problem most of the time. Though incoherent projections are probably the natural state of affairs in all animals, and choirs are likely lacking, there is a simpler way of handling everyday messages. The codes are spatiotemporal firing patterns, as abstract as a bar code, and the distorted version, f(A), reaching the far end will serve equally as well as A (the code space is so enormous that there is little chance of the distorted code hitting upon a code already in use – though, when it happens, you might confuse the sight of an apple with the smell of an orange – so-called synesthesia).

Incoherence is a problem, however, when the receiving cortex wants to send the distorted code f(A) back to the originating cortical area (always via a separate "road" within the arcuate

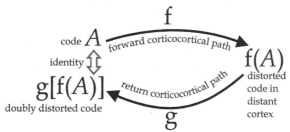

fasciculus, as any given axon is a one-way street). Six out of seven cortical areas have such reciprocal connections. So the apple code arrives back at its origin, doubly distorted into g[f(A)] – not the same thing at all. But no matter, you might reasonably claim: the originating cortex is smart enough so it can eventually learn, with enough repetitions, that the spatiotemporal pattern g[f(A)] means the same thing as A. If A was the code for an apple, f(A) and g[f(*A*)] are alternative codes – it's rather like apple, apfel, and mela (saved by my Italian phrase book) all mean the same thing but in different places. With time spent learning German, apple and apfel bring up the same association – and so it should be with distorted spatiotemporal firing patterns, provided there is time to do all the learning, and provided that the originating cortex can perform this trick with each of the dozens of cortical areas with which it maintains a correspondence (and that means something like *N*-factorial identities have to be gradually established).

There are some real advantages of a common language, a universal code for apple that would work in all places – a sort of Esperanto apple in the brain's various places concerned with apple taste, shape, smell, pronunciation, and so forth. Such a common code would allow novel associations to be formed on the fly, rather than through a laborious pairing procedure. Language is full of never-seen-before associations, such as "a square blue tomato," that you have to work with, passing it around for awhile until some area tentatively responds to it.

DB: This is great! I can see now why protolanguage is so different from true language. When words go to the motor organs of speech one at a time, as they do in protolanguage, lack of coherence isn't a problem – you don't have to join them with other words before you utter them, and you don't have to pass them back and forth. But if words have to be tentatively assembled before uttering them, an incoherent system would change them during the assembly process so that what came out would be just word salad. A common code is an all or nothing thing – you either have one or you don't.

But a common code for apple in even two cortical areas requires coherence in those long corticocortical bundles of axons – which I just said was unlikely on the basis of the typical jumble and fanout in the observed neuroanatomy.

Ah, but anatomy is not destiny – there is a physiological way to recreate the original undistorted pattern, *A*, in the receiving area. And that physiological Good Trick provides a second candidate for the Great Leap Forward, the evolutionary Good Trick allowing syntax to emerge from protolanguage (or, if social-calculus-based argument structure got there first, allowing a great expansion of the workspace that would support many clauses and phrases). Creating order out of incoherence has a critical mass involving a redundancy, not unlike the error-correcting codes used on computer disks.

GIVEN THAT EACH SPATIOTEMPORAL FIRING PATTERN is like a little tune, what my good trick requires is simply a plainchant chorus, all singing the same song. The internal synchronization is provided by the aforementioned axon of the superficial pyramidal neuron, the one whose terminal fanout occurs in a nested set of concentric bands, rather as an express train skips intermediate stops. When the chorus is large enough, and they're all sending axons to the target cortex, you can actually recreate several adjacent instances of code *A* despite the jumble and blur – provided (and this is a theoretical assumption at this time, not data; see chapter 8 of *Code*) that the axon's fanout in the receiving cortex is also a nested set of concentric bands, much like the other axon branches are known to produce in neighboring regions of the sending cortex.

You don't (in my theory) recreate the whole redundant pattern from the sending cortex at first, the way it originally progressed. All it takes is an adjacent pair of hexagons, each containing the unit pattern, somewhere in the jumbled and blurred projection. That pair then seeds the proper melody for what might become a sizeable chorus of *A* in the distant receiving cortical area, a hexagonal mosaic that spreads sideways and recruits new territory. If there is a good resonance for that spatiotemporal pattern in the receiving cortex, the resulting chorus might become even larger than the one that started it from the sending cortex (much like metastatic tumors seed themselves in distant organs).

For any given degree of jumble and blur, there is a critical mass for the sending choir, a number of simultaneous singers (hexagons in the mosaic) below which the receiving cortex cannot reproduce the exact spatiotemporal pattern, not even in a minimal pair of hexagons. And so the distorted spatiotemporal firing pattern, code $f(A)$, has to be used instead, with all its attendant disadvantages for on the fly associations.

RESONANCES TO A COULD BE IN THE SENDING CORTEX alone, with the receiving cortex merely repeating it. Or the sending cortex might be a mere sensory buffer without long-term memory at all; it would send out A to various distant areas, asking their resonances, in effect, "Anyone recognize this?" I did mention, didn't I, that the visual attributes of an apple are likely to reside near visual cortex, that its pronunciation resonance is likely to be near auditory cortex, and so forth?

The cortical area that has a resonance will promptly form up a large chorus singing the song of A, activating similar links to other areas. A successful resonance in one area could trigger the request of the whole cortex's distributed data base; those resonances might contribute the smell of A or the typical pronunciation of A. If all of the relevant regions form up local choruses of A, you get a particularly evocative apple and the word is on the tip of your tongue.

So the concept of an apple is not stored in some particular location; it's best thought of as its universal cerebral code, the spatiotemporal firing pattern A. There are likely local codes as well, A_v, A_p, and so forth, each different because of the contingent history of how we came to learn the sight of an apple, how we learned to pronounce it, and so forth. Each will require an identity with our Esperanto A, the common code for long-distance communication within cortex. At least we no longer need $N!$ identity associations as with incoherent corticocorticals, each slowly learned before becoming useful. The common code A is, of course, equally idiosyncratic – my apple code is surely different than yours – and, I suppose, it's probably closely related to one of the local codes, A_v, A_p, and so forth, perhaps the little tune that first achieved widespread use in other cortical areas.

The nice bonus from this common code is not only efficiency but provisional associations: we can now form novel associations on the fly, as when we first encounter an Italian version of apple pie, proceed to store a resonance for the combination of apple code and pie code, and next trigger it when we again encounter the dish, complete with the link to Villa Serbelloni, identifying where we first tasted it. We can even imagine such a dish, and store the imagined associations.

This is, obviously, not the most elementary way of doing one-trial associative memories; I'm sure that snails learning food avoidance manage without hexagonal mosaics of Hebbian cell-assemblies. But behavior has a time constraint: there are fleeting windows of opportunity. You have to survey the possibilities in a limited period of time and, as brains get bigger and contain more information, that access time may lengthen. Having a common code means you can take alternative paths through the brain to wherever the resonances actually reside in the cortex; there's no path dependence from a series of learned translations of codes, those pesky identities. Just think of the tortuous path that the ancient Greek classics took: Greek to Arabic to Latin to vernacular, with dropouts all along the way because no one was sufficiently interested in preserving or translating a work. That's likely what happens in the neocortex, without a common code from which one-step translations can be done into each modality's working code. When my books are translated, the Hungarian version isn't done from the German, which was done from the Dutch, which was the one done from the original English. Rather than seriatim, they're all done in parallel from a common American English source.

In the case of cerebral sensory and movement modalities, a common code means that a number of routes can be taken from visual to motor cortex, not just one slow route of translation after translation after translation. Each area can translate from the original common code into its local scheme, each can send on the message in the common code – and that's what makes things so flexible and so much better able to handle the novel links needed for the juxtapositions that language tasks utilize.

The common code is often a superposition of codes, with the local area occasionally tacking on another attribute generated from its local resonances. That, Derek, is what I take to be your many-faceted word. A multivoiced symphonic version of the hexagonal code can be a sentence, but let me save that for later, after you discuss the big step up.

DB: Sounds to me like messages in the brain that are not fully coherent are not partially coherent, they are completely incoherent, and with anything less than a coherent message, the brain could not produce a sentence. Is that where you're going?

WHC: Not quite. I'm only saying that the usual incoherent corticocorticals aren't as useful for doing novel associations on the fly. Lacking the speed from corticocortical coherence, you'd make your multiregional connections far too late to be useful for behavioral windows of opportunity.

Recall that I said that a sentence is not just a heap of words, not any more than a house is a mere heap of construction materials? Well, the sentence is really a house of cards, and the breeze that can topple it is called incoherence.

Perhaps I should explain the many uses of the coherence concept, as the term comes with a lot of baggage. (E.O. Wilson also despaired of this and resurrected an old synonym, consilience, for his grand book on how science fits together.) Coherence, outside of the fiber-optics technical context I've been using so far, just means the logical, consistent, orderly relation of various parts. When you use the term more broadly, you're implying that various aspects fit together well, that it "all hangs together" nicely. I might speak of an incoherent memory if I'd confused two people, remembering the face of one with the foreign accent of another.

Incoherence often happens during the initial stages of a memory recall, but we have a "not good enough" detector that keeps us searching our regionally distributed memories until we are confident of our reconstruction of the various scattered parts of the memory. That is, if the situation allows us the time: snap judgements often must be made using still incoherent memories.

Of course, corticocortical coherence in my fiber optic sense is likely to be helpful for preventing incoherent memories. Lapses in neuro-linguistic good-enough detectors would produce incoherent sentences, as the neurologists use the word. But we have to be aware of the dangers of using "coherence" to make analogies between different levels of organization: I've used it at the level of spatiotemporal patterns, Hebb's cell assembly. You can have incoherence at higher levels – say, for memory recall – for reasons other than corticocortical incoherence. Indeed, at a high level, we have a special term for an incoherent result: we "mix metaphors." But such writers are unlikely to have suffered a momentary lapse in their coherence at the cortico-cortical level.

By the way, Derek, you missed an interesting conversation at dinner. At our end of the table, Sontag and I got to talking with the Chinese scholars who are studying the effect of literary translations on modern culture, and we wandered into the problem of translating multiple levels of meaning, how a word-for-word translation would leave a Chinese reader of Joyce's opening words in *Ulysses* missing most of his meaning:

> "Stately, plump Buck Mulligan came from the stairhead, bearing a bowl of lather on which a mirror and a razor lay crossed. A yellow dressinggown, ungirdled, was sustained gently behind him by the mild morning air. He held the bowl aloft and intoned: Introibo ad altare Dei."

What's a poor translator to do? Translating the Latin into local equivalents of "I shall go into the altar of God" gains a little, yet how many readers in China are likely to recognize that it's not only the Catholic mass but a parody of it, tinged with blasphemy? So much of our intellectual task, not just in reading Joyce but in interpreting much of everyday conversation, is to locate appropriate levels of meaning between the concreteness of objects and the various levels of category, relationships, and metaphor. Then often, as when reading Joyce, needing to understand things on multiple levels at the same time.

One of the things that I like best about neocortical versions of a Darwin Machine is that I can easily imagine parallel competitions going on, one at the level of the physical setting (piecing together an old Martello gun tower overlooking Dublin Bay with a full of himself medical student about to shave) and another sorting out candidates at the more abstract level of metaphor (ceremonial words and a deliberate pace – but ungirdled gown and an offering of lather?).

DB: So how do we unite the two interpretations? Another level of abstraction, a superior Darwin Machine fed by both outcomes?

WHC: Not necessarily. Your attention might simply alternate between the two levels, just as it does when driving a car and carrying on a conversation at the same time. If there aren't alternative meldings to consider, that ought to suffice. You don't need Darwin Machines for everything, just novel tasks with a lot of ambiguity.

Indeed, as a task becomes more familiar, the brain handles it differently; for example, an unfamiliar rapid arm movement might utilize the prefrontal cortex on first acquaintance but, five hours later, might primarily seem to utilize the premotor cortex, cerebellum, and parts of the parietal lobe. I suspect that we often find ways to shortcut, using a prefrontalish Darwin Machine approach only when there isn't a more familiar routine to invoke.

I'll bet that analyzing sentences has a number of shortcuts as well, when the subject matter is quite familiar. They might even be more important than the Darwinian competitions, just formed as shortcuts to the Darwinian results from earlier in life.

9

Protolanguage Emerging

We've talked about language and we've talked about the brain. Now it's time to talk about evolution. *What, how,* and now *why*. In the opening chapters, we looked at protolanguage, what it had and what it lacked. But we didn't look at how it had evolved. It was noted that protolanguage bore certain resemblances to the kind of symbolic codes — not real languages, but with some language-like features — that have been fairly successfully taught to apes. But unless we agree with the movie *2001* that our skills and capacities were bestowed on us by aliens from outer space, we have to admit that nobody taught us. Somehow, somewhere, at some time in the distant past — probably at least a million and a half years ago, maybe quite a bit longer — a language system similar to what can now be taught to apes and other brainy creatures must have emerged spontaneously.

Why so long ago? Well, although our ancestors *Homo habilis* and *Homo erectus* were probably closer to apes in their behavior than they are to modern people, they still showed substantial differences from any other primate. They had brains bigger than those of apes, indeed brains that grew steadily throughout the last several million years to a size within the range of modern humans; they spread through a major part of the Old World; they made tools which, though crude and clumsy beside even the tools of Cro-Magnons, were far ahead of anything other species could manufacture; they knew and used fire; they built crude shelters against the weather; and they probably had other skills. Nature preserves only stones and bones, or things that can turn to stone. Artifacts of wood or fiber almost always decay and are lost to us (although recently, in a European bog, long wooden spears with sharpened points that have been dated to half a million years ago were found). None of these things makes it certain that they had protolanguage then but, given that their brains were not that much smaller than ours, it is reasonable to suppose that they did. And don't forget, it's really very unlikely that human language as we know it emerged recently and in a single piece. There must surely have been at least one stage intermediate between no language and full language.

But how did they come by it?

That's the question everyone was asking in the decade or two following the publication of Darwin's *On the Origin of Species* in 1859. What they immediately focused on was the Magic Moment when language began, and they asked such questions as what were the first words like, what did they mean, for what purpose were they created? So much wild and baseless speculation briefly flourished that the linguistic community got turned off on the whole topic of language evolution for the century that followed; even today, most linguists show little interest in it. The focus of those early speculations was unfortunate, for there were many equally interesting and probably more easily answerable questions that could have been asked, such as, given that language got started somehow, how could it have progressed to the complex systems that all human languages possess today?

Probably people then didn't think that question needed answering. Until well into the twentieth century, there was little or no serious study of syntax, certainly nothing beyond long, detailed lists of all the types of clause, phrase, and sentence structure that particular languages used. The big problem seemed to be getting people to talk at all. Once that had been accomplished, it was assumed that language would just naturally get more and more complex.

Nowadays, as subsequent chapters tell, the story of how language got from its birth to its present state is longer, more complex, maybe even more interesting than the story of how language got started. But that earlier story still needs to be told, even if we can't be as sure of the details as we can for the later stages.

WHC: Any theory of cooperation suggests that, as a prerequisite, you have to be able to identify individuals. I'd suggest that unspoken proper names – and particularly for the individuals that you don't see every day – might be a good start for evolving words. Every primate living in a social situation has the problem of identifying the others as individuals, simply because of dominance: does that individual chase me if I don't give way? Or can I threaten him instead? You need to keep track of the state of mutual support among your fellows as well, to judge a social situation – and, as group size increases, the dyads to be remembered rise spectacularly (N!). So proper names are likely to have the conceptual structure there, ready and waiting in the tip of the temporal lobe, for whenever there was the need to make them into words (recombineable units) that were spoken or communicated by stares.

DB: Right, it could be that the naming of individuals was the very first use of words. It's worth noting here the so-called "signature whistles" of dolphins: each dolphin in a pod has a whistle different from that of other pod members, and it seems these whistles are used like names, for identification purposes. But we simply don't know. There's a confusion here that's often perpetuated by people using the term "naming" in an illegitimate sense. They talk about "naming the things in the world" or treat "dog" as a name for "dogs." Most words are simply not names. A name is associated with a particular individual, a word identifies the concept of a whole class of people or things. So getting names doesn't necessarily buy you words. Moreover, apes and monkeys already recognize one another as individuals and indeed have clear maps in their heads that tell them which individuals are related to one another, without any kind of language to help them.

THE FACT THAT LINGUISTS LOST INTEREST in language evolution had no effect on other disciplines. Since the late nineteenth century, scholars from a dozen or more fields have been attracted to the problem. Favored solutions tended, as in many other things, to follow the latest discovery, the latest focus of interest, without always stopping to integrate these things into the broader picture.

Today, the favored explanation for the trigger that set language going lies in the field of social intelligence.

Over the last couple of decades, at least four developments in the behavioral sciences have combined to focus attention on primate intelligence: ethological studies of primates, the concept of "Machiavellian intelligence," theories of "theory of mind," and experimental projects with apes. It's worth a quick look at all of these to see why they made social intelligence seem so attractive as the major selective pressure toward language.

It's hard to remember that forty years ago, all that we knew about primate social life was derived from looking at primates in zoos. This was like studying people in jail and then generalizing to the whole human species. Fortunately, people like Jane Goodall and George Schaller initiated the study of primates in their natural environment, and the result of their pioneering work has been a spate of studies (not to mention shows on the Discovery channel) that have made us almost as familiar with the natural social life of apes as we are with our own. Indeed, the most remarkable thing about ape society is that it does so closely resemble our own. We see the same maneuvering for status, the same family feuds, we see parental and filial affection, the forming and reforming of alliances, altruism, cheating, loyalty, revenge, betrayal. About the only difference between them and us is that we tend to hide our emotions more, bear grudges longer, and accompany all our actions with a torrent of words. Language on top of primate social life is like a mural on a wall – it adds interest and decoration, but it really doesn't change the structure of the wall.

THE SECOND DEVELOPMENT, which arose in part out of the first, was triggered by a seminal work by Nicholas Humphrey. Humphrey asked what selective pressure had served to raise the intelligence of primates above that of other families. The most plausible candidate was social life itself. In the small, tight-knit groups that characterized many (but not all) primate species, there would be a ceaselessly escalating arms race between individuals, each seeking to get the better of the others. Humphrey's work was followed by a series of studies, in the main anecdotal but impressive in their number and consistency, showing acts of calculation and deception on the part of several primate species, which seemed to become more frequent among species closer to us. It seemed as though the tough act of staying successfully selfish within a social community, and competing with individuals some of whom were as smart or smarter than oneself, required a lot more intelligence than, say, hunting or making tools. So, if language was the ultimate flower of intelligence, what more plausible conclusion than that social intelligence produced language?

THE THIRD DEVELOPMENT was a growing interest in what is known as "theory of mind." An age-old philosophical problem is, how do we really know what goes on in other people's minds? How can we tell whether the concepts or emotions or subjective experiences they have are the same as, or different from, those that we have, and to which we all give the same names? One thing we feel sure of is that the *knowledge* in other people's minds isn't always the same as ours. But children aren't necessarily aware of this. One test for "false belief" goes as follows: the child is shown two puppets, call them Bib and Bob. Bib puts some food in a box, then goes away. While Bib is away, Bob moves the food to a second box. Bib comes back. The child is asked, "Where does Bib think the food is?" Most children under four will answer, "In the second box." They know it, and Bob knows it, so why shouldn't Bib know it?

Over two decades ago, the question was raised as to whether other species, in particular other primates, had a theory of mind. Today there is still no clear answer. However, a number of scholars believe that, like language, theory of mind is not an indivisible monolith. One component of a theory of mind is having some idea about what other individuals want or intend. But, as these scholars point out, this is a prerequisite for language as we know it. If someone says, "Isn't it scary in here?" we may know what the actual words mean, but we also need to know whether the speaker is appealing for our reassurance or simply wants us to confess our own fear. And because manipulating others (into, say, getting them to reassure you) or tricking them (into, say, getting them to confess weakness to you) are, at a simpler, nonlinguistic level, things that other primates already do, what more likely than that these competing drives (to trick and manipulate, versus avoiding being tricked and manipulated) constituted the selective pressure that favored language?

Finally, attempts to teach symbolic systems to apes, once their focus had changed from "determining whether apes can acquire language" to "what components of language can apes require?" provided a powerful reinforcement for the social intelligence theorists. If apes already had components of, or at worst, prerequisites for language, what likelier hypothesis than that the demands of competition within small self-contained societies brought these latent characteristics to the surface?

NO ONE CAN DOUBT FOR A MOMENT THAT, once protolanguage had emerged and had reached an appropriate (not necessarily a very high) level of sophistication, it was enthusiastically co-opted for manipulation, deception, enhancement of individual prestige, social grooming, gossip, and all the other functions that social intelligence theorists have rightly assigned to it. In a highly social species, it could hardly be otherwise.

Yet in spite of this, there are good reasons for supposing that the first emergence of protolanguage had very little to do with social intelligence. I'll start with some doubts about a very widespread assumption. One reason for theorists discarding hunting and toolmaking as prime movers in language is that these activities require relatively little intelligence as compared to the demands of a complex social life. Concealed in this claim is the assumption that to start any kind of language requires a lot of intelligence. Once exposed, the assumption looks far from certain. If creatures like sea lions and parrots can be taught symbolic units, then what a creature needs to acquire them spontaneously is surely not so much intelligence as a need to impart concrete information about the real world.

Because that's what language does to perfection, while other animal communication systems can hardly do it at all. Animals can give alarm calls warning of a predator, but they can't say, "Those footprints are a leopard's" – they can't even point to the footprints and say "leopard!" Animals can erect their fur or show other signs of anger but they can't say "I'm angry with you because you cheated me." We may use language most often to flatter people or exchange gossip, but that doesn't tell us anything about why language arose in the first place. By the same reasoning, we could prove that computers were invented to surf the web or play video games. It makes no sense to try to explain language while ignoring what language does uniquely and does best.

Now think about the selective pressure itself. If social intelligence was the driving force behind language, how is it that language has emerged whole and perfect in one primate species and shown not the least sign of appearing in any other? This particular selective pressure must have been shared by all advanced primates except perhaps the solitary orangutan. All of them were competing with one another, conniving, manipulating, yet only we got language. Why us, and not them? Normally, a similar selective pressure will produce the same results across a range of species. For instance, if the climate suddenly cools, hair will get longer and thicker in several species, not just one. Therefore there must have been something special in the human case that did not operate on other primates. What could that something have been?

"More complex social lives" would be a good answer, if the facts supported it. They don't. As noted above, if you take language away, it's far from clear that our social lives are any more complex than those of chimpanzees or bonobos. How would language have increased the fitness of animals who could already handle a rich and varied social life? If there had been no other motive, language might even have been dysfunctional. The animal most skillful in using it might have given away too much about itself, might have provided a more taciturn rival with information that could then have been used against it.

An increase in group size is another possibility that has been suggested. But there is absolutely no evidence that group size among hominids one million or two million years ago was any greater than group size among bonobos or chimpanzees. On top of which, it's not clear that group size is a criterion of anything. Human hunter-gatherers and chimpanzees both have what are called "fusion-fission" societies – their group size fluctuates as they divide into small groups and then periodically come together again in larger groups. Which group size is the right group size?

SO THE SELECTIVE PRESSURE FOR LANGUAGE had to come from something that was unique to hominids and something that required the exchange of factual information. Let's think for a moment about hominid ecology and how it differed from that of apes, ancient or modern. Apes live mostly or entirely in heavily forested regions of the winterless tropics. The frequency of trees and the ability of apes to climb them better than any potential predator put apes virtually beyond the reach of effective predation. What this means in terms of their daily life is that they don't have to devote the time and energy that many creatures do to the business of watching for and evading predators.

Chimpanzees aren't strict vegetarians by any means, but in the tropical regions from which they have never succeeded in escaping, they can usually find enough fruit, nuts, or leafage to satisfy them. Meat is a rare luxury. They can usually locate an adequate supply of food without going very far. In the course of a day they may not wander outside of an area of a square mile or so.

On both these counts – predation risk and food availability – the lives of early hominids were very different. Instead of tropical forests, they inhabited grassy savannas with isolated stands of trees and what are known as "gallery woods" – those narrow, winding woodlands, only a few trees wide, found on the banks of rivers in savanna areas. There one couldn't be sure of a tree to run up, or of success if one did, as there's an obvious tradeoff between bipedal walking and the ability to climb trees. It would do a modern human little good to try climbing a tree if pursued by a leopard, for instance. We don't know how quickly or how gradually that tradeoff occurred, but we do know that our ancestors started walking on two legs at least a million years before any serious brain enlargement, so they were probably relatively poor tree climbers by the time even protolanguage emerged.

Moreover, savannas were, as they are today, prime predator country. Outside comic books, the lion is not king of the jungle; indeed what you notice most about tropical forests is that there's very little life on the ground and therefore nothing to attract predators in off the savanna — whereas on the savanna they find great hordes of herbivores just asking to be devoured. Indeed, there were many more predators (and more different species of predators) around two million years ago than there are today, including some much bigger and more fearsome than those of today. Our ancestors of two million years ago, however, were much smaller than we are. Yet, just like us, they lacked the natural offensive weapons — claws, big sharp teeth, high speed over short distances — that are the weapons of choice for savanna predators. A species so ill-equipped would soon have gone extinct if its members hadn't devoted far more time to predator detection and predator avoidance than apes do. But predator detection and predator avoidance depend not on social intelligence but on what we might call "pragmatic intelligence": the noting and interpretation of clues in the environment (footprints, crushed vegetation, and so on), something that apes don't seem to have.

Then there's the question of food. Unless you're adapted to eating grass — one of the few things that hominids weren't adapted to eat — there really isn't much food in savanna country, and what little there is comes in a bewildering variety of forms. There are a few trees and bushes here and there that yield fruit or nuts or berries, but because these are widely scattered and only bear for short periods at different times of the year, you have to remember what's in fruit, where and when, if you're not going to have many wasted journeys. You can't just wander around thinking you're bound to stumble on something sooner or later. There are roots that you can dig up and eat if you know what the plants growing out the top look like and whether they are poisonous or not. There are eggs or fledglings in the nests of ground-nesting or shrub-nesting birds, which are usually well hidden and which, apart from stumbling on them, can only be located by carefully watching and correctly interpreting the behavior of parent birds. There is the honey in the nests of wild bees that is delicious and highly nutritious, but extremely hard to get at without painful and possibly fatal consequences. There are small terrestrial animals, particularly the young of these, which, if you are skilled in observing and interpreting the traces they leave, you can sometimes kill with a thrown stone or by running them down. There are fish in the rivers and pools which, even before the invention of hooks and nets, you could, with immense caution, creep up on and catch by hand (at least, one of my wife's uncles could, and surely any non-tool-using foraging skill accessible to effete modern humans must have been within the reach of our remote ancestors). There are the carcasses of dead animals of varying size, locating of which is easy (especially if you are watching the vultures) but which immediately puts you into direct competition with other, more powerful and better equipped scavengers. (Remember that the old dichotomy between scavengers and predators has been broken down by recent studies – any predator will scavenge if the bodies are there, just as any scavenger will predate if the prey can be caught fairly easily.) All these many and varied food sources were not conveniently located in an ape-sized terrain and continuously available, but scattered thinly over dozens of square miles of terrain and three hundred and sixty-five days of every year.

WE TEND TO THINK OF OURSELVES as continuations of modern apes (you can always get a feature article out of asking, are we more like the aggressive, opportunistically carnivorous chimpanzees or the less aggressive, more sensual bonobos?). Modern ethology has given us a picture of ape social groups spending many hours just lollygagging about, like modern humans at a holiday camp, teasing, grooming, play fighting, having a whale of a good time. It's easy to imagine things have always been that way. We assume too often that the common ancestor of chimps, bonobos, and us was something pretty much like a modern chimp or bonobo, maybe halfway in between, and that the others more or less stood still while we changed radically.

But this view of things may be wide of the mark. The common ancestor of our little primate subfamily is believed to have lived between five and seven million years ago, and modern apes may be as different from the apes of three million years ago as we are from australopithecines.

WHC: The so-called competitive exclusion principle suggests that the extant apes might be the ones that avoided direct competition with our ancestors, for example, that the gorilla survived because it retreated into a vegetarian niche. Chimps and bonobos may not be perfect stand-ins for our common ancestor, but the many social behaviors that we share with them (see Frans de Waal's books) suggest that we're seeing ancestral behaviors, not ones separately evolved in the last five million years.

Unless you believe that ecology, the environment, and the way animals get food have no effect whatsoever on a species, you have to believe that in important ways, we were different long before we talked, maybe even before we walked upright. A lot of typical ape behavior would have had to be suppressed, or at least severely curtailed, under the conditions that early hominids experienced. Now that our niche allows them, now that our control over nature is complete enough to give at least some of us the necessary leisure, we can give free rein to those social behaviors, and indeed I've been told that the idle rich spend whole lives on them. But to say that because we do something now, and apes do it now, and our common ancestors did it, therefore at every stage of our evolution we must have done it – that's saying the environment doesn't matter in evolution, only genetic inheritance counts. I'm sorry, that's only half the evolutionary equation. The environment does matter. Interaction between animals and environment is what evolution's all about.

SOCIAL LIFE DIDN'T GET MORE COMPLEX for our remote ancestors; what did get more complex was the interaction between our ancestors and their environment. Increased wariness, increased curiosity, a far greater and more ruthless concentration on the exigencies of getting a living – these must have been the qualities that most sharply distinguished early hominid life, and that paid off most in terms of procreation and perpetuation of genes. Bonding, and the reciprocal altruism that cemented bonds, would of course have remained vital – you would want to be sure that, in a confrontation with predators, your buddy stayed by you or at least covered your retreat by throwing stones. But the strongest selective pressures would have come from the brute exigencies of survival. If we want to look for the pressure that first set language going, we must therefore look at the kind of life early hominids lived and the kind of behavior that this life would foster.

One can tell two possible stories, one involving foraging and another involving instruction of the young.

The foraging story goes as follows. Either the group foraged as a single unit or split into smaller units to forage. If they split, the story is straightforward. If one unit discovered an abundant food source that could feed all of them for a day or two, how would they tell the other units this? In other words, how could they evaluate competing food sources? That problem doesn't go away even if the group foraged as a single unit. Remember that our ancestors had to be a lot more aware of their physical environment than arboreal apes.

Now suppose the group has just found a store of honey and is exploiting it, getting stung in the process. One member happens to look up and sees vultures circling just above the horizon. There's dead meat there, maybe some dead megafauna that would feed the group for days. He jumps up and down, pointing. They're too busy with the bees and the honey to take any notice. What's the advantage to him if he can get their attention? If he's right, and they make a big food find, he'll be a hero, the others will look up to him, his status in the pecking order (and his access to mates) will be substantially enhanced. If he does this sort of thing consistently, he may get to be the leader. But how can he make them understand? If only he had a real word or two, something more specific than follow-me!

The instruction story goes like this: A mother and her young child are walking along a trail. The mother sees a footprint, which she identifies as that of a leopard. The little girl is running past without a look. How can the mother prevent a scenario in which, before experience can teach her the connection between leopards and footprints, the bearer of her genes runs happily past the footprints and into the jaws of the leopard lying in wait in the tall grass? She can point, we may suppose.

But pointing out the footprint is barely half the story. The larger half is explaining what it means. And how can you do that without words? If only she had just the one word!

Now of course these are just-so stories, and we all know that just-so stories are just that: stories. What's wrong with them, it's claimed, is that you can make up a just-so story for any scenario you can think of. Or so they say. To date, nobody that I know of has produced a just-so story for the social intelligence theory of language origin. That is, nobody working within that particular framework has suggested what the first symbolic utterances might have

> WHC: But Derek, that's easy (as long as great specificity isn't required). The Gombe chimps simply use the vocalization *Wraaa*! ("That's weird, get away from that!") Even unspoken spookiness is quite sufficient to be passed down through a few generations. Every time I hear one of those elephant stories —you know, the ones about the herd still avoiding the road where great-great-grandmother was shot a few generations ago —I am reminded that "superstitious behavior" works very well for such things, juveniles copying their elders, and so on for generations.

meant, and under what circumstances they would have been uttered. The point here is that anything, even the crudest and most limited form of protolanguage consisting perhaps of a handful of words and/or gestures, has to have had an immediate payoff for the individuals who used it. If it didn't, the behavior wouldn't have continued, certainly wouldn't have gotten fixed into the genotype. Nobody doubts that social uses of language (or protolanguage) would have paid off enormously in terms of individual fitness, but it seems to me that before they could do that – before our ancestors could say even simple things like "I like you" or "You got nice eyes," let alone "If you and I fight together, we can lick Alpha," or "Your favorite female cheated on you with Beta this afternoon" – linguistic ability would have already gone well past its starting point.

However, it's easy to imagine what the first symbols might have been in either of the stories I told just now. In the first, something like "Mammoth! Mammoth!" (which could have been the noise the beast made, or miming a trunk, or anything that worked) plus "Come on!", which might have been repeated arm movements in the direction of the circling vultures. In the second, something like "Leopard!" (however that was rendered) plus pointing at the footprints and perhaps then raising a finger to the lips to indicate silence and caution. But so far, no supporter of the social-intelligence theory has come up with anything comparable. I'd be interested to see them try.

There's one important corollary to the instruction story. One of the most interesting findings about Kanzi the bonobo is that, like human children, he engages in pretend play. Kanzi "enjoys feeding a toy dog imaginary food" or "may pretend that a toy dog or toy gorilla is biting him"; he asks Sue Savage-Rumbaugh to pretend to be a monster and chase him, and pretends to be afraid of her, although it's fairly obvious that he isn't. It's risky to generalize from one individual to a species, especially if that individual's upbringing is as untypical of bonobos as was Kanzi's. But it does raise the possibility that pretend play is genuinely homologous, and that accordingly we may suppose that the children of hominids engaged in it. If they did, then there can be little doubt that those children took the symbols they learned from their elders and incorporated them into their play, experimented with them, and expanded them. The relative plasticity of children's brains and their capacity to both learn and innovate are not the be-all and end-all of the language story, but they may well have contributed significantly to it.

THIS CHAPTER IS, I KNOW, LARGELY SPECULATIVE, and may never be proven or disproven. But nobody knows how much we may yet be able to learn about our remote ancestors. If we do learn more, it won't be just a question of amassing facts. We can't do without facts, but facts by themselves, alas, never say enough. All facts are subject to interpretation, and can take on completely different appearances depending on the lens through which they are viewed. Speculation forms a vital component in science; it helps to interpret facts and to guide future research, but if the research it has guided turns up things that it didn't predict – even things quite incompatible with it – that's par for the course. Provided you don't turn the goal into a religion, you get more out of looking with a goal in mind than out of blind fishing expeditions. Speculation is light luggage, it's easy to junk it and try again.

At present, we still simply don't know enough about the Magic Moment of the first symbolic utterances to be able to do more than speculate. Short of cloning *Homo erectus* from bone-marrow found in frozen bogs, which is still science fiction but might not always be, we will never know for sure what its linguistic capacities were. In the unlikely event that an erectus gets cloned in my lifetime, I'd like to be the one that gets to give it language tests. I'd predict that around age two or less it could be taught protolanguage and that it would be more inventive than apes have been, but that attempts to teach it true human language would fail dismally. If it did learn syntax, a lot of this book would need re-writing. If it didn't, and couldn't learn, it would go a long way to confirming the picture presented here.

Meantime, one or two things indirectly support that picture. Most of the first fifty words any child learns are nouns, just like the "Mammoth!" and "Leopard!" of our just-so stories. Not hello, goodbye, please, thank-you, or any of the expressions you might predict if language had arisen to cement social networks. Words like these are used very frequently in children's presence and are often actively modeled for them at an early age. "Milk!" "Say *please* Sally!" "Milk!" "No, Sally, say, 'Milk, please!'" "Milk! Milk! Waaa-a-a-a-ah!" How many conversations like that have we heard, or even participated in! Indeed there are societies in which almost the only verbal interaction adults have with children is to teach them the niceties of polite discourse, the right way of talking to aunts, cousins, grandparents, and so forth. None of this seems to make much difference to what children learn first, which is a set of labels they can attach to salient objects in the world around them (or more exactly, to their concepts of such objects).

So, I would argue that the deepest roots of language will be found to lie in extractive foraging or the instruction of children, rather than in social intelligence – important as that intelligence was as a prerequisite for language. To be motivated to communicate information, you have indeed to be able to think, in some form, "I know X; Y doesn't know X; I should gain Z by telling Y about X." But that doesn't mean that social intelligence was the pressure that pushed us, and us alone, out of the infinite host of alingual species into a minority of one.

———————————————————————

WHC: Apropos your observation that hominids were not limited to spoken words: words could be expressed via distinctive postures or starring (and apes are quite good at picking up on what another is looking at), with vocalization versions added later. For example, pointing might be added when the distances are so great that others cannot see what you're starring at (Kanzi, by the way, started pointing when only a year old). Vocalizations are handy when darkness or line of sight (often a problem in dense forests) limits the usefulness of starring and pointing. Indeed, the region surrounding the sylvian fissure is even more related to hand-arm and oral-facial gestures than it is to vocal control, judging from the exposed cortical surface identifiable with a function.

The lift of an eyebrow might have expressed an early verb, with direction of gaze identifying the individual concerned, and a hand posture simultaneously communicating an adverb. Pairing novel vocalizations (ones not part of the exclamation repertoire) with such gestures might have been the way that meaningless phonemes got their start, as supplements to a nonvocal gestural repertoire. Then, as vocal fluency improved, spoken words might have displaced gestural equivalents.

I like your evocation of what it must have been like to make a living on the savanna with the anatomy of *Homo erectus*. I know what various paleoanthropologists say about hunting, and I think that it is focused so narrowly as to miss the big picture; when the history of anthropology is written, the denial of hunting's role is going to be seen as very odd. It's difficult even now to understand why a much-needed explication of gathering roles in evolution was exaggerated into a denial of the importance of hunting.

The gathering-is-more-important fans then seized upon tooth- and cut-mark evidence for scavenging to say, in effect, that if our ancestors ate meat, it was only because it was already dead. But chimps seem not to scavenge (they don't consume dead monkeys left on a path for them to discover), though they sure do hunt. Scavenging is, in any event, a top-of-the-food-chain niche that can only support a very small population; still, it could have been of importance in a transition to successful hunting. I certainly understand the tendency of archaeologists to focus on the "hard evidence" they can find in the

East African Rift Valley and emphasize behavior that's related to it.
But why ignore major facts about hunting? Let me list a few:

Most obviously, there's the exquisite throwing accuracy of modern
humans compared to that of apes. (Would paleoanthropologists prefer prehistoric baseball to hunting, as an
evolutionary explanation for accuracy? Flinging is surely a
prime defense, to fend off those other savanna predators, but
even chimpanzees fling branches.)

Once hominids expanded out of the subtropics, there's a little
problem from an annual period of plant dormancy, technically
known as "winter"; though grass remains nutritious in winter,
pre-agricultural humans likely preferred to eat animals that
ate the grass during the few months when gathering was
made difficult by snow and frozen ground.

Then there's that half-million-year-old wooden spear that Derek
mentioned. (Would they prefer prehistoric javelin contests to
hunting?)

Most recently, there's that paleodiet evidence from the isotopes
that suggest the more recent hominids were eating a lot of
grass, either directly or indirectly. (As much as I like bread, I
suspect it wasn't directly.)

Chimps chase and consume small monkeys and piglets; kills are so
prized that they will temporarily disrupt the prevalent dominance
hierarchy; high-ranking males will beg for a handout from a low-
ranking possessor, rather than simply snatching the prize. (What
theoretician of social life would dared to hypothesize such a bizarre
thing! And think what the critics would have said. Still, it's true.)

[Besides intensification of function and increased efficiency, there is] another entirely different and much more dramatic way by which evolutionary novelties can be [acquired is via] a change in function of a structure. Here an existing structure, let us say the [sensory] antennae of *Daphnia*, acquires the additional function of a swimming paddle and, under new selection pressure, become enlarged and modified. The feathers of birds presumably originated as modified reptilian scales serving for heat regulation but acquired a new function on the forelimbs and tails of birds in connection with flying.

During a succession of functions, a structure always passes through a stage when it can simultaneously perform both jobs.

–ERNST MAYR, 1997

10

Reciprocal Altruism as the Predecessor of Argument Structure

I'm about to do something that at first sight may seem paradoxical and perverse. I spent a chapter claiming that social intelligence had nothing at all to do with the emergence of language. Now I'm going to claim that syntax, which I and others see as *the* distinguishing feature of human language, derives from one of the most important components of social intelligence. What's going on?

The only reason my moves might seem paradoxical is because people don't always distinguish clearly enough between the emergence of protolanguage and the emergence of syntax. These are two entirely different things, even if one did eventually lead to the other. If I'm right, the events weren't even close in time. It's not only possible, it would have been pretty easy for a species only just ahead of the other apes to get along with words (or signs – makes no difference) and nothing else for a million years or two. Evolution is a conservative thing. It doesn't need constant novelty. Good enough is good enough. At least, until something better comes down the pike.

So there's no inconsistency in proposing that, although social intelligence had little to do with the birth of protolanguage, it had a lot to do with the birth of syntax. But I might as well warn you, the story of how syntax came to be is not a simple one, not the kind you can boil down into a thirty-second soundbite. To follow it, we'll have to follow a long

> The greatest thing
> You'll ever learn
> Is how to love
> And get your love right back
> —ERUTAN YOB

and tortuous trail, through social intelligence, the birth of altruism, cheating, episodic memory, and then on into some aspects of how the brain works that definitely don't form part of *Brain 101*. So we might as well start with sex.

SEX GETS PEOPLE'S ATTENTION. And of course it's central to evolution. It makes us procreate, and procreation leads to variation, and variation is necessary for natural selection; otherwise there'd be nothing to select from. As if that weren't enough, differential interests in sex (males want to spread their seed as widely as possible, females – who do the real work – want to limit their offspring to the best and brightest) drive a great deal of animal behavior. Female preference for particular types of mates determines many creatures' physical form and behavior (peacocks' tails, bowerbirds' bowers, battles between rutting stags, and on and on).

We modern humans tend to forget, when we pursue our romantic inclinations with little restraint beyond the willingness or otherwise of our prospective lovers to cooperate, how lucky we are in comparison with a number of other mammalian species. Take bull elephant seals, for example. In each troop of these masses of blubber that can be seen decorating the Californian coast, the largest and most aggressive male (the alpha male, as ethologists would call him) virtually monopolizes the females in the group. Any male seal who wants to break this monopoly has to choose a moment when the alpha male's attention is otherwise engaged. If not, his first move in an amorous direction will be met with extreme physical violence. No matter how receptive a female bull elephant may be to the advances of another suitor, a head-on charge from an alpha male discourages all but the most reckless. It has been estimated that up to 85 percent of all copulations in a group are performed by the alpha male. As there are several other mature males in each group, this means that large numbers of male elephant seals mate extremely rarely and indeed some of them may go to their graves as virgins.

This arrangement may be advantageous to elephant seals as a whole, as it ensures that only the toughest and brawniest pass on their genes to succeeding generations. But then again it may not. Brawn's fine, but what about brain? Does the sexual dominance of alpha males help make elephant seals smarter? Probably not. Certainly elephant seal brains are tiny relative to their immense body size, and they show no sign of doing much beyond lying on rocks and catching fish.

Smarter species are unlikely to put up with forced celibacy if they can find a way to escape it. And the easiest way, perhaps the only way of dealing with a member of your group who is stronger than you, is to form an alliance against him. Two heads are better than one, and so are two bodies and two sets of teeth. A pair of medium-tough monkeys can take on any alpha male.

Unfortunately, there's still no direct evidence of a correlation between forming alliances against alpha males and reproductive success. There is, however, a correlation between neocortex size and both frequency of tactical deception and the social skills involved in competition between males. That's to say, in species with bigger brains, the sexual tyranny of alpha males is typically circumvented. Because those species are precisely the ones in which male-male alliances are formed, this does provide some indirect evidence that the motive for alliance formation is primarily the desire to spread one's genes.

TWO ANIMALS WHO FORM AN ALLIANCE against the alpha animal are not necessarily kin. Yet recent research does seem to indicate that while an animal may do things that help to perpetuate its own genes (and hence may help close kin, who carry a proportion of those genes), it doesn't, normally or naturally, do things that will benefit some set of competing genes. (Nothing mysterious about this – if there had been animals that gave the genes of others preferential treatment to their own, those animals would surely be extinct by now). So how could altruism have developed? Only if helping someone else indirectly helps you – if, when I scratch your back, you scratch mine.

And that's how reciprocal altruism, father of the more selfless kinds, was born.

The term was coined by biologist Robert Trivers. For a long time people had puzzled over the existence of altruism among humans. Why were some of us willing to sacrifice our own interests, occasionally even our lives, for others? This question became even more pressing with the rise of Darwinism, the decline of belief in the supernatural, and a growing acceptance that all living organisms are of their nature irredeemably selfish.

As Trivers showed, and as many subsequent ethological studies confirmed, reciprocal altruism was the answer. You may wonder how selfish behavior could spawn selfless behavior. But even the cynic must admit that, on occasion, humans do sacrifice themselves for others, even for members of other species, without hope of reward. That kind of altruism has a slightly different story, a story mediated by language and featuring duty, responsibility, and ideal forms of behavior. (It would take us too far from our path to tell that story here — we should merely note that this broader type of altruism could never have come about if the more self-oriented types had not preceded it.)

But wait a minute, you may say. What do you mean by saying "take us too far from the path"? Aren't we a long way from the path already? What on earth have elephant seals and sex alliances and reciprocal altruism to do with language?

AS A MATTER OF FACT, reciprocal altruism contains the roots of many of the things we hold most dear — morality, democracy, and yes, even language (or at least syntax). For the morality and democracy bits, you should read Frans de Waal's delightful (and extremely important) book, *Good-natured*. Nothing we could say about them would improve on that.

That anything as abstract as syntax should have come from reciprocal altruism may well seem surprising. For what I'm proposing here is that the practice of reciprocal altruism created the set of abstract categories and structures that, once they were joined to a structureless protolanguage, yielded the kind of syntax that all modern human languages exhibit.

Consider what primate social life was and is like. Primates character-istically live in small groups, seldom exceeding a hundred individuals or falling below a dozen or so. In other words, these groups are small enough for each individual to know every other individual quite intimately. Primate social life, as many excellent studies vividly show, is an intense and continuous experience. Individuals are competitive, flexible, and opportunistic; they won't succeed if they don't keep on their toes. Alliances based on reciprocal altruism play a vital part in helping individuals to succeed. Describing a troop of baboons, Shirley C. Strum observes that

> Friendships were almost formal systems of social reciprocity. The underlying understanding seemed to be, "If I do something good for you now, you'll do something good for me later." The balance sheet would be set up in an individual's favor by a combination of good deeds and hard-won trust. This was quite a sophisticated process when one took into account the time that might pass between credits and debits. A new male coming into [the troop] acted as if he had thought to himself, "To be successful in this troop, I'll need a few female friends, several infant friends . . . and some male allies." He would then set out to acquire them. Weeks, even months later, he would call in his dues.

As this extract shows, the building of such alliances takes time, and exploiting them to the full takes more time. It places a heavy load on the memory, too, if you have to remember over weeks and months who you owe and who owes you.

Alliances will not last without constant work to maintain them. You cannot use someone to gain your own ends and then just ignore them. You'd feel used if you were treated like that. And the more you learn about primates, the more you appreciate that their emotions do not differ substantially from ours.

One vital factor in group cohesion and bonding between individuals is mutual grooming. Primates of many species spend hours examining one another's hair, far more time than would be justified if the practice was no more than a means for removing parasites. Although any group member may groom any other, members of alliances groom one another much more frequently than non-allied animals. But in any alliance, the question must be: does A groom B much more frequently than B grooms A?

All of us have been, at one time or another, tempted to cheat – to give in return less than we have received. Cheaters may be gross or subtle. Gross cheaters accept your favors and do nothing in return – they're easy to spot. Subtle cheaters are another matter:

> A subtle cheater reciprocates enough to make it worth the altruist's while, but returns less than he is capable of giving, or less than the altruist would give if the situation were reversed.

How can you recognize a subtle cheater? Cheaters, subtle or otherwise, must be unmasked, for if cheaters can get away with it, who will fail to cheat? And if everyone cheats, then the system of reciprocal altruism breaks down into a war of all against all.

So it must be possible for any member of an alliance to detect whether his partner is cheating or not. If neither partner is cheating, the alliance can be maintained indefinitely. If one partner is cheating, then the other is wasting valuable time and effort that could be better spent on a different partner. Animals with partners who don't cheat will do better (suffer less stress, win more fights, gain more sexual access, and thus probably leave more progeny behind) than animals whose partners cheat and get away with it. If animals originally fell into two classes (good cheater detectors and not so good ones), then over long periods of time, the good detectors would gradually squeeze out the poorer ones. Good cheater detection would then form a fixed part of that species' genetic recipe.

So it should be possible, in any species that typically practices reciprocal altruism, for animal B to know whether he grooms his partner A more or less often than A grooms him. And grooming, although it's among the most important primate activities, is by no means the only activity in which reciprocal altruism comes into play. Take meat-eating among chimpanzees, for example. Chimpanzees, like many human hunter-gatherers, like to hunt young monkeys as a valuable source of protein; this practice probably goes back to the common ancestors of chimps and humans, if not earlier. In general, chimpanzees do not share food, but when one or two of them kill a monkey, they share the meat with most chimps that beg hard enough for a piece.

There is a good reason for this. Successful hunts, unlike finds of fruit or nuts, do not happen every day. Because they are such rare occurrences, even a successful chimp would go a very long time without meat if meat wasn't shared. Chimpanzees share food for the same reason they carry out any other act of reciprocal altruism – if they didn't, they wouldn't get the benefits they otherwise could.

And so it goes. In addition to remembering who groomed who and how often, who gave meat to who and how often, chimpanzees and other primates have to keep track of how often partners stood by them in fights, how often they ran away, and doubtless other types of behavior too. In other words, to detect cheaters and protect their own interests, they are obliged to develop a social calculus that weighs their own acts against the acts of others.

WHAT WAS NECESSARY FOR SUCH A CALCULUS? It would require at least the following ingredients: (1) an ability to distinguish individuals of the social group, (2) an ability to distinguish different types of action, and (3) some kind of abstract representation of the roles of participants in actions.

The first is essential because you have to know who's who before you know who to form alliances with, and that's a prerequisite for any kind of reciprocal altruism – even for the one-off "I-just-did-something-for-you-so-now-you-owe-me" kind, let alone for the stable alliances that characterize so much primate social life.

The second – distinguishing different types of action – is essential because if you can't distinguish, you can't keep track of whether you are doing favors for your partner more often than your partner is doing them for you. But wouldn't it be simpler if you just had a single category called "Actions requiring reciprocity"? After all, the nature of the actions isn't relevant, all that matters is making sure the balance stays in your favor. Well, just try to imagine how you could possibly set up such a category in the brain. It's too vague, too abstract, too general. On the other hand, many primate species – not just apes, but even some monkeys, such as macaques – have assemblies of neurons that respond to particular actions, like some other primate grabbing for them. If individual actions can be represented in the brain, and if some are already represented, it shouldn't be too hard to set up the mechanisms for telling whether you did X to someone oftener than someone did X to you.

The third feature – distinguishing roles of the participants – is essential because reciprocal altruism isn't like a kinship system, where a given individual always has the same relationship to others. Sometimes you are grooming, sometimes you're being groomed. Thus the categories have to be abstract enough to cover a variety of individuals, each of whom will perform the role concerned at different times. Roles like AGENT (the performer of an action) and THEME (who- or whatever undergoes the action) will then serve like tags, to be attached to any individual whose role, on a particular occasion, happens to fit.

Now consider episodic memory. The exact status of episodic memory remains somewhat controversial. But although the relationship between episodic and semantic memory may be uncertain, nobody doubts that humans have the capacity to remember events in the order in which they occurred, and remember too, for most events, who or what performed the action and who or what it was performed upon. Some believe that episodic memory is shared by many species. If it is shared by other primates, then we can suppose that every time primates record an event in memory, they tag each participant in that event with the role of AGENT, THEME or GOAL (whoever the action was directed towards). Thus they too, when they remember the event, will remember exactly who did what to whom.

With the apparatus I've described, you can keep track of individuals, remember how often they've done things for you and how often you've done things for them, see whether there's any imbalance there, and determine whether that imbalance goes against you. (I can't imagine monkeys lying awake worrying over whether the imbalance went the other way, whether they had done enough for others, but a more conscience-stricken species could use the calculus for this too.) In other words, with that apparatus you have a mechanism powerful enough to detect cheaters and freeloaders and make reciprocal altruism really work as the lynchpin of your social life.

WHC: You've persuaded me that what reciprocal altruism (RA) needs, besides identification of individuals, is some mental bookkeeping for debts: "I supported Alpha the last time he was challenged by Beta, so maybe I can get away with taking this morsel of food, after all." From such beginnings, a concept of debt could have later developed: "Alpha owes me."

But when do debts need to be communicated, in ways beyond the body language that signifies reluctance to re-engage in sharing or supportive behavior? A vocalization for "But you owe me!" would be an interesting public way of labeling an individual as a freeloader. (I don't like the term "cheater" – it implies an implicit promise to reciprocate and that's a bit fancier a concept than we need here, like using adultery when promiscuity would suffice.) If such a cry reduced the tendency of other individuals to cooperate with the individual so labeled, it would have some force in evolutionary terms.

RA, after all, is not going to get started with an explicit set of promises of reciprocation. It's more likely to be a matter of mutual grooming or food sharing with individuals until a significant imbalance arises, then reproaching the other or withdrawing from further cooperation. From a sharing foundation, coalitions might develop that would subvert the usual dominance hierarchy.

Getting started down the RA path requires individual identification, an ability to categorize advantageous acts (and who they advantaged), a memory for the balance of debts, some level of an indiscriminate tendency to share (to get things started), and a sufficiently rich environment so that the occasional losses are not serious compared to the rewards of cooperation (grooming, food, sex, dominance). There might be a hierarchy of cooperation: mutual grooming is cheap, food sharing less so, and support in conflicts likely to develop only upon a successful foundation of other cooperation because of the risks of being bitten or losing dominance rank while actively assisting another in a chase or fight.

Altruism has always been mixed up with the whole issue of group selection. About thirty years ago, many people turned their backs on group selection because it looked, mathematically, as if freeloaders could always swamp the boat – that even if you had, by chance, a subpopulation form up with a high percentage of individuals having a genetic tendency to share, or to perform other altruistic acts (say, breaking up fights between unrelated individuals, risking injury to do so), the situation wasn't stable: it would always deteriorate as the freeloaders received more than they gave back, diluting the altruistic genes because their reproduction was enhanced. It wasn't an evolutionarily stable strategy.

Trying to see the "big picture" can mislead you. In this case, there were several errors: aggregating all subpopulations together to talk of a grand average, and focusing on what's stable in the long run without taking into account what shorter-term fluctuations could generate via pumping.

First, suppose that inbreeding subgroups with altruism out-reproduce subgroups that lack it. Yes, even though those altruistic groups are going to backslide in the long run, they can still – in the short run – raise the overall percentages of altruism when such a group expands faster than the other groups. And it's not just a mathematical abstraction: allow the subgroups to merge into one big group, and the altruistic genes are more than before the prior split into separated subgroups. So the overall short-term picture can look very different than the long-term one, if only populations split occasionally into subpopulations and later merge.

The notion that group selection "can't work" always reminds me of what intellectuals said about the second law of thermodynamics a century ago. Literary types from Swinburne to Henry Adams knew all too well what the second law said and reasoned that if heat flows invariably from hot to cold, that the stock of useful energy in the world is always running down, and that disorder (so-called "entropy") is always on the rise, therefore the universe is moving toward "heat death."

Of course, a closed system like the universe may exhibit rising levels of disorder while, at the same time, local pockets of order are arising. Open systems like the Earth, with enormous throughputs of energy from the Sun, have a tendency toward self-organization, the same as you can see in a pan of cooking porridge if you fail to stir it (the surface becomes furrowed into cells, even hexagonal mosaics on occasion). So too, populations made up of many inbreeding subpopulations can exhibit local pockets of successful altruism.

Second, the long term may never arrive, because the climate changes in the meantime and pumps up the fading percentage with another round of selection favoring groups with more altruism. Beware of the combination of aggregation and of long-term thinking, or you may miss seeing the interesting stuff, all those good stories.

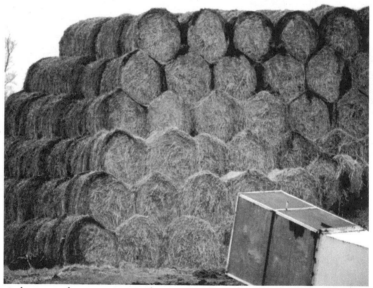

Order arising from compression: hexagons in a haystack, near Cambridge, England. (photo by Dan Downs)

11

Role Links for Words

I would be the last person to suggest that the social calculus described in the preceding chapter was the only thing causing representation of thematic roles in primate minds. Other factors have surely contributed to the same end. But if you think about it, only the social calculus could have built up categories that had the right degree of clarity and abstractness.

If you understand what causes things you may be able to predict them. Accurate prediction may save your life. Saving your life gives you more time to procreate, so current evolutionary thought suggests that prediction should be favored. If you know that movements of long grass when there is no wind may be caused by a predator stalking you, you can take appropriate action in time, rather than passively awaiting the tiger's charge. But are we to suppose that the genes code for every eventuality, and abstract across categories as diverse as moving grass and falling rain? Or is it more likely that each animal has to learn the consequences of these things from its own experience?

I suspect that the answer may lie somewhere in between: that nothing so specific as the detection of tell-tale grass swirls is hardwired, but that prey animals have vision that responds to things like movement in grass, and also mechanisms that tell them that something is causing that movement and that that something is a predator. Nothing here needs to incorporate an abstract concept of agency. All the information is specific to that one kind of event.

However, we're not talking about one kind of event. We're talking about a variety of events – grooming, food sharing, chasing, fighting – in which any one animal is sometimes the performer, sometimes the object of the action. (Sometimes it's me grooming you, sometimes you grooming me, sometimes a third party, and so on.) When all of this takes place among animals of a high social intelligence who need to keep track of one another's behavior to avoid being shortchanged by freeloaders, it would hardly be surprising if some quite abstract analysis of the roles developed.

What I think happened was that the social calculus set up the categories of AGENT, THEME, and GOAL, and that these categories (or *thematic roles,* which is what linguists call them) were then exapted to produce the basis for sentence structures. Some linguists might object that thematic roles are semantic, and syntax is, well, syntax. Syntax is autonomous, a totally self-contained country with its own rules and regulations, and ever more shall be so. But I think here that the linguists are ignoring the nature of evolution. It's like saying, well, swim-bladders were a floatation device, and lungs are for breathing, so lungs can't have evolved from swim-bladders. However, we know that they did.

Nothing in evolution is a complete novelty. Everything is a modified version of something that came before – even if the modification sometimes changes the original past recognition. So, syntax could not have emerged as a pure novelty. But there was semantics before there was syntax, and if some aspect of semantics could be expressed in terms of syntax, then that aspect makes a prime suspect for the source of syntax. What happened to it afterwards is another matter.

What matters now is not so much the semantic nature of the roles themselves. What *was* important was getting the primary roles of GOAL, AGENT, and THEME represented in the primate mind. It didn't have to *go on* being important, once the function of those roles diverged, once they were exapted to play a part in language. The really important thing is that those key roles *had* to be expressed in sentences:

▷ With a verb like "sleep" or "run," you have to express one role.

▷ With a verb like "make" or "break," you have to express two.

▷ With a verb like "give" or "persuade," you have to express three.

In other words, you know in advance, in every clause of every sentence depending on the clause's verb, whether you will have to be looking for one, two or three noun-phrases to which these roles are attached — that is to say, for one, two, or three "obligatory arguments."

I have assumed throughout, for reasons discussed at length elsewhere, that language began in the form of a structureless protolanguage, something like an early stage pidgin, without any formal structure — just handfuls of words or gestures strung together. Syntax began when people began to map thematic roles onto their protolinguistic output. What this means is simply that when they talked about anything that had happened, they would put in the obligatory arguments. Instead of saying things like "Ig take," they would have to say "Ig take meat," even if everyone knew it was meat they were talking about. Instead of saying "hit Og," they would have to say "Ig hit Og," even though everyone knew it was Ig who had done it. And once they knew what had to be there, they could go on to longer and longer sentences, for the following reason.

An argument is simply the combination of a thematic role (AGENT, etc.) with whatever words represent a participant in an action, state or event. More often than not, those words take the form of a noun-phrase (remember, we call it a noun-phrase even if there's only a single noun or pronoun there). But they could just as easily be a whole clause, because what an argument actually is depends on the verb. If the verb is "break," then its THEME is going to be some hard physical object that might conceivably be broken ("He couldn't break the lock" is fine, but "He broke the blanket" is the kind of sentence you get from little kids who haven't yet learned the verb "tear"). But if the verb is "say," then its THEME is going to be anything that can be said, including clauses that could, if they stood alone, be sentences in their own right. Thus, in "He said he was tired," the clause "he was tired" is just as much an argument of the verb as is the noun-phrase "his prayers" in "He said his prayers."

THEY SAY THERE'S NO FREE LUNCH, but here's an exception. However long a sentence is, you can always make it longer, thanks to recursivity By mapping argument structure onto utterances, you get recursivity for free. And recursivity is one of the defining characteristics of true language – it's why sentences can be infinite, why Faulkner's 1,300-word sentence can never be the longest English sentence, why there never can be a longest English sentence.

Recursivity should be distinguished from mere iteration. *Iteration* looks like

$$1 + 1 + 1 + 1 + 1 .....$$

Recursivity looks, for anyone who may be familiar with obsolete versions of generative grammar, like this:

$$S \Rightarrow NP\ VP$$

[A Sentence can be rewritten as a Noun-Phrase and a Verb-Phrase]

$$VP \Rightarrow V\ (\ NP\ )$$
$$(\ S\ \ \ )$$

[A Verb-Phrase can be rewritten as a Verb and
(optionally) a Noun-Phrase or even a Sentence]

What this means is that units at higher levels of structure (like NP and S in the first line) can be reintroduced at lower levels, so that the process of sentence building simply recycles and recycles for as long as you want it to. It's recursivity that gives language its wonderful flexibility, allowing us to introduce several ideas into the same sentence, let them brush against one another and strike sparks – the sparks of novelty and creativity that form the most distinctive feature of our species.

Updating the old generative formula, recursivity now looks like this:

$$AS \Rightarrow V + A_1 (+A_2 (+A_3))$$

[An Argument Structure can be rewritten as a Verb
plus one, two, or three Arguments]

$$A_i \Rightarrow NP/PP/AS$$

[An Argument can be rewritten as a Noun-Phrase,
Prepositional Phrase, or Argument Structure]

However, this formula still lacks an important element that the old formula had: *linearization*.

LINEARIZATION IS NOT something we wanted. It was something that was forced on us by our choice of a physical medium for language. When we speak, we use only a single channel, the vocal channel, and we can't make more than one sound at a time. If we'd chosen sign, we could in principle have produced two or three units simultaneously – even though this possibility isn't exploited as much as it might be in the sign languages of the deaf. But with the vocal channel we're stuck with one sound after another, one word after another. Thus, sounds and words have to be linked in some definite order, and that means word order becomes one possible means of resolving ambiguities and indicating structural relationships.

To many, especially those who are not syntacticians, word order looms large in syntax. To some, it's the be-all and end-all. Once words have been arranged in a fixed order, they think, we're done. Far from it, for several

> For every complex problem, there is a simple, easy to understand, incorrect answer.
> ALBERT SZENT-GYORGYI

reasons. First, even in English (a fairly strict word-order language, as languages go) you can put the same words in any number of orders – "Mary made the video," "The video was made by Mary," "It was the video that Mary made."

And secondly, the really crucial relationships in language are not horizontal but vertical (whether something is higher or lower in a tree diagram of a sentence, whether a particular tree branch includes or doesn't include a particular item, and so on). Horizontal linear relationships can't explain why "Bob's sister hurt herself" is grammatical but "Bob's sister hurt himself" isn't. They can't explain why "How do you know who left?" is grammatical but "Who do you know how left?" isn't, even though the corresponding statement, "I know how Mary left – by Yellow Cab" is fine. They can't explain why the subject of "work for" in "Bill wants someone to work for" is "Bill," while in "Bill wants someone to work for him" it's "someone." And these are just three randomly chosen examples out of countless thousands that horizontal relationships can't explain and vertical relationships can.

However, you can easily get from an abstract map of argument structure to a linear string by starting with the verb and adding arguments to it in a certain order. This order isn't set in marble (we can monkey about with it, even in English, as the "Mary and the video" examples showed). But there is (in English at least) an order we can take as basic. Interestingly enough, this order is the basic order that we find in creole languages worldwide, and because the original creole language speakers didn't have a fixed word order in their input, it's a fair bet that this order is the most natural among all the variants.

First, if there is a GOAL argument, this is attached to the right of the verb, followed by the THEME argument, which is attached to the right of Verb + GOAL. Then, if there are any optional arguments like TIME, they are attached to the right of Verb + GOAL + THEME. Finally, AGENT is attached to the *left* of everything else. In other words, if you have a sentence like

Mary gave Bill a watch last week.

it's built up in the following stages:

gave Bill	[Verb + GOAL]
gave Bill a watch	[Verb + GOAL + THEME]
gave Bill a watch last week	[Verb + GOAL + THEME + TIME]
Mary gave Bill a watch last week.	[AGENT prefixed onto verb phrase]

When there's no GOAL, then THEME moves up next to the verb, but nothing else changes:

> Mary kissed Bill.

When there's no AGENT, then THEME moves up into its vacant slot:

> Mary dreamed.

The same thing happens if you want to tell a story from the perspective of Mary, or if you don't know (or don't care) who the AGENT was:

> Mary was kissed [by Bill].

Once you know this much, you can really start to parse and understand complex sentences.

LET'S LOOK AT AN EXAMPLE OF HOW THIS WORKS in practice by comparing it to protolanguage limitations. First imagine you're a proto-language speaker and somebody has said something like

> I saw Og taking Ug's meat.

Well, not exactly that, because before there was true language, it's highly unlikely that there were things like past tenses or -*ing* forms or apostrophe -*s*. So it would probably have come out more like "I see Og take Ug meat." How could you have parsed this?

Well, you couldn't. You might have got to "I see," with a small problem about whether the speaker had seen, would see, or was seeing right now. But then you would have been confronted by "Og," and you would have no way of telling whether "Og" was the THEME argument of "see" or the AGENT argument of "take," or both. The third option, both, would have helped you to understand the sentence better, but it's the least likely to be chosen, because in protolanguage, words are in one place and do one thing and one thing only. A speaker familiar with protolanguage would have been far more likely to assume that either the THEME of "see" had been omitted (so "Og" would be merely AGENT of "take") or that the AGENT of "take" had been omitted (so "Og" would be the THEME of "see"), because that's the kind of thing that happens all the time in protolanguage.

But this is nothing compared with "Ug meat." No surprise to find two nouns together (this happens all the time in protolanguage) but their relationship is up for grabs, even with the verb "take" around to help out.

Could it mean that Ug was taken to the meat, or from the meat, or the meat was taken to him, or from him?

Now there's no doubt that an intelligent protolanguage speaker could eventually, with the help of context, of knowing the people concerned and their behavior, have figured out the correct meaning. But life goes by too fast to allow us the luxury of sitting around trying to figure out the meaning of every six-word sentence, and there will always be times when we fail. We need something automatic, like what we have in language today. Let's see how, with our modern equipment, we might get to understand

I saw Og taking Ug's meat.

even without all the -ing's and s'es and so on that we nowadays have to help us.

The first verb is "see." We know that "see" needs two arguments. "I" as AGENT of "see" precedes it and is easily identified. The THEME should follow it, but the word immediately following it, "Og," is then followed by another verb, that also requires a preceding AGENT. The alternative conclusion is that the THEME of "see" is all the rest of the sentence – a reasonable conclusion because what one sees can be a situation or event just as easily as it can be an object. Now all we have to do is look for an AGENT of "take" ("Og," obviously) and a THEME of "take." Since "take" is a two-place and not a three-place predicate, we know there can't be two more obligatory arguments, so again the plausible conclusion is that "Ug meat" is a compound phrase of the type "possessor-possessed."

The precise identification of this last phrase is the only thing that could give us trouble. What tells a modern speaker the relationship between the last two words is, of course, the apostrophe "s" ("Ug's meat") that marks the first noun as possessor of the second. And that's just one example of grammatical morphology – all the words (and things smaller than words, inflections and the like) that don't refer to real-world entities, but indicate relationships between entities (like "to," which gives the idea that things change places), or more formal relationships between different bits of the sentence (like the "s" on present-tense English verbs that tells you their subject is third-person singular).

Notice that even the functions that don't relate to formal structure tell us things about that structure. An apostrophe "s" on a noun indicates part of a genitive (possessive) construction. "The" signals that the rest of a noun-phrase will follow it – we know not to look for any part of that noun-phrase to the *left* of "the." As markers of structure, and in particular of boundaries between phrases and clauses (not all, but many grammatical terms serve this function), all of these things help us to parse and understand sentences. They don't put an end to ambiguity – we don't know, unless explicitly told, whether "I saw the boy with the telescope" means "I saw the boy who had a telescope" or "I used a telescope to see the boy." But they reduce ambiguity to an acceptable level.

WE'VE LOOKED AT HOW SYNTAX WORKS when we're parsing and comprehending sentences. Now let's see how it works in production. In the epoch of protolanguage, the impulse codes that represented words were presumably dispatched one at a time to the motor control areas controlling speech. Once the social calculus had been mapped onto protolanguage, things would have changed. If the brain happened to come up with a verb, the regions where nouns and verbs were stored – the temporal and frontal lobes – immediately started talking with one another.

Say the verb was "kick." The frontal lobe called up the temporal lobe, so to speak, and said, "Hey, this needs two arguments, so send me up an AGENT and a THEME, a kicker and a kickee." Say the temporal lobe sent "girl" and "cat." Quick as a flash, the frontal lobe started to fit together first "kickcat" and then "girlkickcat." If you want to know when this started happening, let's say maybe 150,000 years ago.

Nowadays, of course, it's a bit more bureaucratic. Before being incorporated, nouns now have to be checked with the memory store to see if the hearer ought to know what you're talking about; depending on the result, you'll get either "a girl" or "the girl." Verbs before being incorporated have to hook up with morphemes that indicate things like number and person and tense, adding things like "*-ed*" to make "kicked", so the message that finally arrives at the motor controls of speech is whatever sequence of signals that spells out "thegirlkickedthecat."

This is probably *not* how you think that you say a sentence. You likely think that you first have a thought, something like <THE GIRL KICKED THE CAT>, and then you find words to fit it, "The girl kicked the cat." But that's just your conscious mind's imaginary reconstruction of something you can't possibly have experienced, and is probably about as accurate as our naïve inference about the sun going around the earth. What actually happens is something much more complex and chaotic than what I described in the previous paragraph.

The thing that you think you deliberately and consciously decided to say is, however, simply the winner in a Darwinian competition between it and dozens of other things, some of similar meaning, others quite different, that you might have said instead. The parts of your mind that deal with language are incessantly bouncing words and phrases about, whether you want them to or not. If you don't utter them, they still appear in the form of inner speech, that James Joycean internal monologue that, when you try to meditate, or sleep after a hectic day, you find almost impossible to turn off. Even sleep doesn't turn them off entirely; they go on to script the dialog in your dreams.

BEING HUMAN, WE LIKE TO FOOL AROUND with our language. Precisely because this template of argument structure remains forever in our subconscious minds, we can afford to fool around, if only within strict limits and in pretty specific situations. For instance, I can omit THEMES after certain verbs ("Bill's eaten already," "Mary sang nicely"). But what do you suppose Bill ate? Coal? Sawdust? And did Mary sing an aria or the New York phone directory? Obviously what they ate or sang was something edible or singable, and if the kind of food or song doesn't matter, you needn't mention it. There are quite a few verbs like that, verbs that have implicit arguments like "write" (what else can you write but words?) or "drink" (what can you drink but liquids?). Or take "They played golf." "They played tennis," "They played together." Nobody is going to think that "together" is some new game they hadn't heard of before. When you acquire syntax, you don't lose words, and the meanings of words will clue you if someone takes liberties with regular syntax.

In addition to leaving things out, we can put things in. We're not limited to just the thematic role(s) that a verb specifies. We can add in optional ones, so long as they're drawn from the very short list available: PLACE (the only other role that's ever obligatory, and that only for a tiny handful of verbs like "put"), TIME, BENEFICIARY *(doing something for someone)*, INSTRUMENT *(doing it **with** something)*, SOURCE *(taking it from someone or something)*. Maybe there are one or two more thematic roles – you can get into arguments with linguists (who will argue about almost anything) over exactly how many roles there really are, but there are very few and I've mentioned all the important and common ones.

But, you may say, all this is predicated on the supposition that things start with a verb – that your brain throws up a verb first and then pulls out things that can carry the thematic roles specified by that verb. Suppose it started with a noun, wouldn't that mess things up?

Not at all. Probably what's driving your train of thought (if you can call it that; it's more like a bunch of Roman chariots racing toward the finish line, jockeying for position, each one trying to knock others out of the race) is the memory or imagination of some complete episode, so that if a noun comes uppermost, it drags the verb of an accompanying action with it.

> WHC: That is, by the way, the verb test that I said (p. 25) made the brain area in front of your left ear work so much harder, compared to merely naming the noun.

Even without an episode to hold things together, there's no problem. A very common psychological test involves giving subjects a noun and then asking for a verb that goes with it. Try it on your friends. If you say "bicycle" they'll probably say "ride," if you say "knife" they'll probably say "cut" (if they say "stab", watch them carefully). If they say "cut" for "bicycle" or "ride" for "knife", or if they just gawk at you, you can assume they're brain-damaged in some way.

There are very fast links between verbs and the nouns they habitually associate with, links that can work in either direction.

So far, we've pretty much stuck to nouns and verbs and skipped all the other stuff – the articles and prepositions and particles, not to mention the inflections of nouns and verbs that add information about number and tense. Where do all these things come from?

Well, they're totally absent from ape "talk", and extremely rare, if present at all, in early pidgins and toddler talk. In other words, they're absent from varieties of protolanguage. And this is exactly what you would expect if one of their major functions is that of signaling structure.

BUT, AS POINTED OUT ALREADY, argument structure on its own can't remove all the ambiguities from syntax. And so, in the millennia that followed the birth of syntax, our ancestors must have been competing with one another to produce devices that would make that syntax more readily parsable, hence easier to understand automatically.

This means there would have been Darwinian competition, with the best and the brightest trying all manner of ways to disambiguate the ambiguous sentences as economically as they could. In other words, *the newly emerged syntax would itself have acted as a selective pressure,* tilting the balance in favor of any changes in the nervous system that would lead to the construction of more readily parsable sentences. The consequent adaptations would have improved the fitness of individuals, because those who could get their points across better would have tended to occupy leadership roles and thus gained access to a wider selection of mates. All it takes in evolution is a marginal edge, and if you have it, sooner or later your genes will replace those of others who don't.

WAIT, YOU SAY, ISN'T THIS DISCREDITED LAMARCKISM, the belief that what you do in your lifetime can somehow get into your genes? Not at all. It's a form-follows-function principle known as the Baldwin effect.

James Mark Baldwin, a late nineteenth-century psychologist, pointed out that changes in behavior could change selection pressures. For instance, in the words of one authority on Baldwin, Robert J. Richards,

Some ground-feeding birds that happened to enter a new swampy terrain might learn in each generation to wade out onto a pond to feed off the bottom. Those that were flexible enough to acquire such responses would survive. In time, congenital variations might begin slowly to replace acquired traits, with natural selection molding them into instincts for wading and pecking at the right-sized objects. So what began as learned behavior and acquired modification might in time become innately determined and part of the hereditary legacy of the species. Organic selection [Baldwin's own name for the Baldwin effect] thus imitated Lamarckian inheritance but remained strictly neo-Darwinian.

What happened next in the evolution of syntax most probably followed along these lines. Once our ancestors had changed their behavior by producing complex sentences, a varying aptitude for developing means to make those sentences easier to understand would have come under the automatic and irresistible pressure of natural selection. Those children who could accomplish, spontaneously and automatically, what their elders could only do by conscious and difficult effort —produce devices for disambiguating sentences – would have had a leg up on their less well endowed competitors in the social competitions. There may have been many different devices at first. The way evolution normally works is to throw up all manner of possibilities and then let competition thin them out. We can be fairly sure that what we find today represents the cream of whatever crop there was then.

Don't get me wrong, though. What got fixed was definitely not *particular* markers – words with a specific shape and

WHC: Not necessarily the 'cream of the crop' of early devices , Derek — not any more than VHS was better than Betamax, or Windows was better than the Mac's operating system. Sometimes you just standardize on something that is merely "good enough." In economics, they talk of "market capture." The best doesn't always win, because not everyone can afford to stay in the game.

sound for marking tense or structural boundaries. What got fixed was that there *had to be* specific markers for such things. Children came to expect them and look for them. And if they didn't find them – if, for example, they received input from a primitive pidgin – they put them back in. If you want to know the formula for what turned out to be the most favored solution, check it out in the appendix.

In other words, what I formerly conceived as a single step from proto-language to true language can be broken down into two stages, one of exaptation (the core phrase-and-clause producing argument-structure machine) and one of Baldwinian evolution (adding mechanisms useful for marking the new structures with grammatical morphemes and making them more readily processable). These Baldwinian universals simply formed part of the cascade of change that was triggered the moment that the syntax engine started running: a cascade that included more rapid neural processing, clearer and faster articulation, as well as other ambiguity-reducing devices.

HOWEVER, THE NEED FOR GRAMMATICAL MORPHOLOGY to mark unit boundaries and other features meant that the language had to produce new words and inflections (which probably started their lives as full words, see below). These words had little if any referential meaning. (What does "of" mean in "the discovery of America" except "Look out, this noun phrase doesn't end with 'discovery'"?) Where did they come from?

Well, for a typical example, look at what happened in Tokpisin, a new language in New Guinea that's often called a pidgin but has been a creole since World War II. Its earlier pidgin form had only "him" as third-person-singular pronoun, regardless of position – "Him catch him," for example, though "catch" came out sounding something like "kis." The second "him" got reduced over time to lightly stressed "im", so that speakers began to hear it as attached to the verb that preceded it. Soon it lost its meaning as a separate pronoun and just meant something like, "Wait, a THEME argument is coming next." Simultaneously, things were kept acoustically and perceptually separate by changing the form of the third-person-singular pronoun to "em." So "he catches him" is now "em i kisim em", which looks like "him he catches him him" but isn't, of course (the "i" is just another grammatical marker that means, "Look out, a verb is coming next!").

We can only suppose that the earliest true language did the same as modern creoles have done: took content words from the prior protolanguage and bleached and downgraded them, first into free grammatical morphemes, then into mere inflections. Most contemporary creoles have yet to reach the final stage, but the whole cycle has been experienced by many, perhaps all older languages.

But, you may say, surely protolanguage had some grammatical morphemes. What about words like "in" or "on" or "to" or "from"? Surely they would have needed words like these just to find their way around and tell people where things were.

We've suggested that protolanguage most probably arose out of extractive foraging. Whether it did or not, extractive foraging must have been one of the major uses to which protolanguage was put. In the last few years, biologists, ethologists and anthropologists alike have so focused their attention on the social life of primates, they seem to have forgotten that primates had to eat. And because, in order to eat, they would almost certainly have foraged in small groups and reported back to the main group, they would have needed to be able to give directions and describe locations as well as tell what kind of food could be found at the end of the trail.

But how do you arrive at something as abstract as an "on" or an "in"? Again creoles give us clues. In a number of these languages, the preposition corresponding to "on" comes from a noun meaning "the top." The preposition corresponding to "in" comes from a noun meaning "the inside." The preposition corresponding to "under" comes from a noun meaning "the bottom," and so on. In Guyanese Creole you often hear an expression that sounds like "a road kaana." If you recognize the third word as the local pronunciation of "corner," you will assume this means "at the corner of the road." Wrong. It actually means "by the road" or "beside the road." The "a" is a general locative/directional particle that just marks the optional thematic role PLACE, and the noun "corner" is turned into a postposition (that's just a preposition coming after, instead of before, the noun) equivalent to "beside."

So it's quite likely that the original protolanguage got nouns that meant "top," "bottom," "side," "corner," and so on, and that when the syntactic engine came along, these came in handy both to mark the thematic role PLACE and to distinguish the various kinds of PLACE where things might be. Indeed, if you look at creoles, you can find examples of every kind of grammatical morpheme a language might need, all produced by this process of bleaching and downgrading content words. If modern humans can do this kind of thing, why not our ancestors of a hundred-odd thousand years ago?

THIS CHAPTER HAS SHOWN how a protolanguage could be turned into a full language by a single exaptation followed by a series of Baldwin effects that any such exaptation would be bound to bring in its wake. But I'm sure a rather obvious question has been bugging you for quite some time now.

I've claimed that protolanguage has been around for maybe as long as two million years, and that a social calculus has been around for a lot longer than that. So how was it that, when protolanguage first emerged, the social calculus didn't immediately get mapped onto it to give us syntax and modern language a couple of million years ago? Why was syntax *delayed*?

This puzzled me for a long time, in fact until I talked to Bill. Then I knew that what he proposed just had to be right. So I'll let him explain it to you.

12

The Word Tree as a Secondary Use of Throwing's Segmented Movement Planner

Derek,

So far as I can see, your social calculus predecessor has the fire power needed to do most of role links, and they could be enough for comprehending a recursively embedded sentence. But I can suggest a step up in efficiency that might make a structured sentence a frequent occurrence rather than a slowly created affair dependent on learning.

Because my step has a critical mass, somewhat like your full glass that finally overflows with additional drips, it might well provide a flowering of structured thinking and structured language, the sort of improvement in higher intellectual function that might have produced the great surge in technological and artistic innovation seen during the last ice age – but not in the prior two dozen ice ages, when brain size was enlarging.

While I suspect that categories can be stored almost anywhere, let me assume that the temporal lobe rearrangements are one physical manifestation of the great expansion of words. There would probably be a lot of social-calculus-style role links associated with the proper names stored in temporal tip, or with the facial expression recognition that is another known specialty of temporal lobe.

152

I'll also assume that the frontal lobe is the site where proto-language's simple utterances are planned – premotor and prefrontal (that's the frontal lobe in front of premotor) are the areas most obviously involved in planning novel movements of all sorts, so perhaps they planned protolanguage utterances as well. Judging from its connections to midbrain for the rapid orienting responses, the frontal lobe might also be the home of those closed-class words that express relative location (*above, below, in, on, at, by, next to*) and relative direction (*to, from, through, left, right, up, down*).

Even if protolanguage didn't utter orienting words, hand movements might often be associated with them, as can be seen in modern Italy. Their use as markers of the boundary of a phrase might have followed, much as my pidgin Italian substitutes hand motions for a forgotten word. And because the frontal lobe tends to be involved with planning, perhaps the closed-class words for relative time (*before, after, while*, and the various indicators of tense) also live there.

So if you want a dichotomy, let me suppose for a moment (this is, of course, an oversimplification) that nouns and adjectives are mostly temporal lobe and that verbs and boundary words are mostly frontal lobe. Even a simple sentence requires their interaction, in this simplification. How does temporal lobe interact with frontal lobe, you ask, to intensify the style of sentence planning? Is there something about that interaction which might provide the Great Leap Forward, when our ancestors finally got their language act together?

DB: That makes a lot of sense from a linguistic perspective. Traditionally, the four major word classes – that is, nouns, verbs, adjectives and prepositions – have been distinguished by assigning to them plus and minus values of the two major categories, noun (N) and verb (V) as follows:

Noun	+N	−V
Adjective	+N	+V
Verb	−N	+V
Preposition	−N	−V

In other words, adjectives are both nounlike and verblike, and prepositions are neither. So for good linguistic reasons, linguists made exactly the distinction between adjectives and nouns (both +N) and prepositions and verbs (both −N) that the brain does.

Back in our early days at the Villa Serbelloni, Derek, you challenged me to come up with a neural mechanism for the step up from protolanguage to using syntax. I replied that I could actually think of a possibility, nicely illustrating how things might have happened. Here's a better version of what I was trying to say that day, as we sat outside on those park benches on the terrace, back in the humid heat before the postcard-clear autumn days arrived. And now I have the additional benefit of those ideas from our third week in Bellagio, when it became evident from playing bocce how the argument structure from the social calculus could have helped retrain the frontal lobe's segmented planner you use for "get set" in throwing, for use as a word tree.

NEUROPHYSIOLOGISTS DO COME AT the language problem from a slightly different angle than most of the linguists do, who are often happy if they can just explain how a sentence might make sense. To me, part of the answer also has to involve the preparatory background to that sentence, the process you use to generate alternatives and make decisions between the better candidates. It's not enough to explain the structures for making sense of a completed long utterance; you also have to explain the "little person in the head" that generates the ideas and comprehends the input. Otherwise, you wind up with Dennett's fallacy of the stage on which scenes are played out for some viewer.

And that dualism isn't far from the point of view taken by the 1977 book that formed my first introduction to the Villa Serbelloni, *The Self and Its Brain.* In 1972, the philosopher Karl Popper and the neurophysiologist John C. Eccles participated in a conference here in Bellagio on reductionism in biology. They must have liked it because, in September 1974, the two of them returned to hold a series of conversations here, sitting out on this same terrace and listening to an earlier generation of roosters crowing, down the hill in Pescalo. Their talks featured some top-down attempts by Eccles (otherwise, very much of a bottom-up neurophysiologist whose Nobel Prize-winning spinal cord work in the 1950s formed the background for my more humble Ph.D. thesis on spinal cord neurons in the 1960s) to find the interface between his brain and his (very Catholic) immortal soul.

My neocortical Darwin Machine suggests one way that the little-person-inside problem could be avoided, as a Darwinian process provides explicit accounts for creativity, comprehension, subconscious thoughts, and for how attention might shift from a present topic to a new one, all without a central stage, with all the dynamics described in 1880 by William James:

> Instead of thoughts of concrete things patiently following one another in a beaten track of habitual suggestion, we have the most abrupt cross-cuts and transitions from one idea to another, the most rarefied abstractions and discriminations, the most unheard-of combinations of elements, the subtlest associations of analogy; in a word, we seem suddenly introduced into a seething caldron of ideas, where everything is fizzling and bobbing about in a state of bewildering activity, where partnerships can be joined or loosened in an instant, treadmill routine is unknown, and the unexpected seems the only law.

But might the Darwin Machine also support – or even explain – syntax, that great aid to structured thoughts of length and subtlety?

THE NOTION OF COMPETING SOLUTIONS tends to orient you toward explanations that will allow an entire candidate sentence, complete with embedded phrases and clauses, to be compared against another complete candidate, with all its own phrases and clauses also in place. Yes, you may earlier have one phrase competing against an alternative phrase, but you also have to have a way of judging a complete sentence for its quality relative to another candidate sentence. You also need to judge the winner against internalized standards for solutions "good enough" so that you can finish, moving on to something else (otherwise, you send it back for further revisions).

But the production problem for structured sentences is far more difficult than the comprehension problem. How, I asked myself, could one possibly judge the whole sentence against alternatives and standards as one prepared to speak? That would involve having to unpack the winner into the motor program needed to pronounce the words in the right order. It had, I saw, to embody a two-level approach, something like the linguists' distinction between deep structure (whether argument- or phrase-based) and the surface structure conventions of the particular language.

DB: We should really clear up this whole business of deep structure and surface structure, because this terminology has passed into the public domain of interdisciplinary discourse, and everybody uses it, regardless of whether or not they understand it. If they don't understand it, they can now cop to that without losing face, because the distinction's mythical. We've come a long way, baby, but we've come round in a circle.

No, that's not quite fair – we've come round in a huge sweep just like the path here in Bellagio that circles the hill where the Villa stands. You suddenly find yourself directly above the place where you were ten minutes ago. You haven't made any linear progress but you're way up above where you were and the vista is immense, you can see where you are, how you got there and where you're going, which you couldn't before. So couldn't linguistics have short-cut it, you may ask, scrambling directly up the hill instead of wasting thirty years on this detour? Maybe, maybe not. At places here on the hill in Bellagio there are huge cliffs that you couldn't hope to climb. The only way to the top is round about and up. Maybe the last thirty years in linguistics were like that.

Don't take my word for all this. Take Chomsky's. Yes, in his latest (post-1990) minimalist model, Chomsky has finally removed the distinction, which he himself created, between deep and surface structure. There is now just one level of syntax, which is a "projection of the lexicon." What this means is that, in the dictionary of your own language that you carry around in your head, stored in the distributed patterns of neural resonances that Bill's told you about, there is stored along with each word all the features of that word. The features of a word (which form part of what we've been calling the role links) include its meaning, its number and gender (if it has any), the word-class or classes it belongs to, its function (if it's a grammatical morpheme), the thematic roles it assigns (if it's a verb), and so forth. Some of these features take the form of requirements: for instance, the article "the" requires a noun-phrase after it, the auxiliary verb takes only a present or past participle after it (you can say "is speaking" or "is spoken" but not "is speak" or "is spoke") and so on. What then happens is that you try to merge words to make larger units – phrases and clauses – by matching features. If the positive features of one match the requirements of the other, you can merge them, and move on to the next merger. If not, to use the latest jargon, "the derivation crashes" – that is, you get a spoonful of word salad.

Now this model is a lot closer to how the brain really handles language than the old one. It made no kind of neurological sense to say that the brain first shaped up some very abstract sentence structures and then fooled around with them to make something completely different come out of your mouth, which is what the old deep-structure/surface-structure model was implicitly claiming. Brains aren't that subtle. If they can do it the straightforward way, they do it the straightforward way.

Notice too that at the same time we can get rid of another idea about language that bedeviled discourse for many years. The old model implied that you had to have in your head actual knowledge of the grammar that you had to use to crank out the deep structures (to "generate" them – which was why it was called "generative grammar"). But this knowledge was supposed to be innate. For years, philosophers and psychologists yelled and screamed at one another about whether there could be innate knowledge or not. To try and break the deadlock, Chomsky actually invented a new verb, "to cognize," which means to know something you don't know you know, but it never really caught on.

Controversies like that are never resolved – someone just pulls the rug out from under them and they disappear. Now all that's left of the mountains of innate knowledge the old system presupposed are a few bare principles. And these principles are merely a metaphorical way of looking at what actually happens. The brain acts as if it obeyed such principles, but what it's actually doing is simply executing algorithms for putting sentences together and understanding them once they've been put together. And what this book's all about is how these algorithms came to be.

The planning level needed, I thought, a way that the winners of the regional competitions for each component clause and phrase could, like the voices of a symphony or choral work, combine to produce a totality, one that could compete as a whole with other such wholes. The winning totality would then be decomposed in an appropriate order, rather like a reverse-order version of Benjamin Britten's *Young Person's Guide to the Orchestra* where each voice performs separately, then in combination. The readout for speech is a big problem as you must decompose your symphonic combination and do it in an understandable order – for example, Derek's expected ordering of arguments for the particular language you are currently speaking.

THROWING PROVIDES A NICE EXAMPLE of two levels, namely the distinction between a plan and its unpacked execution. The current group of scholars and artists at the Villa Serbelloni, after a long day of work, tend to drift downhill to the bocce court on the waterfront for a preprandial game or two. The only problem is climbing back uphill afterwards, a little matter of 86 meters (I checked the topographic maps). It's like a tall building, with the dining room on the 25th floor and no elevator (but then another excellent dinner restores us).

Bocce is a European game played on a long, flat court; solid balls (about the size of a grapefruit or softball) are rolled toward a small target ball. The idea is to come the closest to the target ball – or, if all else fails, to move the small ball or the competition's balls by hitting them with a pitched ball of your own. You've got two problems: throwing straight at the target, and not throwing too fast or too slow. Getting your ball to stop in the right place is the hard part of bocce because you must carefully regulate your hand's velocity up to the moment of launch. Beginners always overshoot.

It's difficult because rapid throwing, hammering, clubbing, and kicking are all ballistic movements; that is, once you get the motion underway, you soon pass a point of no return. Your arm can't be stopped; you can't even alter its trajectory. If your shirt sticks to your sweaty arm and tugs a little as you pick up a cup of tea, you have lots of time to correct your arm trajectory before the tea spills. But in the ballistic movements, you can't correct for the disturbance because there isn't enough time for the sensory signal to travel into the spinal cord, up to your brain, influence a decision, and then travel back down to the spinal cord and out to the arm muscles. That round trip takes about one-eighth of a second, and a typical dart throw is over and done by then. You have to make the perfect plan as you "get set" to throw, then put it into execution.

FOR AN UNDERARM THROW, SUCH AS USED IN BOCCE, motions are generated in easily identified segments. The slowest is the forward motion of your upper body. Then there is the rotation of your upper arm around your shoulder, which moves the elbow forward. But, riding atop that, there is another motion being generated that rotates your lower arm about the elbow. Then there's the independent rotation around the wrist and, finally, the loosening of the fingers that let the ball fly free when it has reached the right velocity (not too fast, not too slow).

Because this isn't a standardized throw (as we try to make dart throws and basketball free throws), our "get set" task is to discover a multijoint solution that will launch the ball with the velocity that we judge appropriate to the target's distance (another difficult task, but I'll assume here that it is perfectly done). There are a number of launch combinations that will suffice (fast shoulder and slow elbow, minimal shoulder and a wrist flick, and so forth), but there are millions of wrong solutions to avoid. Still, Darwin Machines are very good at discarding the nonsensical and shaping up the quality of "4 out of 10" solutions into "score of 9" solutions.

But the multijoint aspect suggests that the Darwin Machine's planning task is structured, each joint's movement depending on the others. Were only body forwards motion to be used with a stiff shoulder and arm, the hand cradling the ball, then you could accelerate your body to the right velocity with your legs and then slow down – whereupon the ball would fly out of its cradle. The launch velocity is simply the hand's peak velocity.

With a stiff upper and lower arm and cradled ball, the launch velocity is a function of body velocity and the angular velocity of shoulder rotation and the distance from shoulder joint to the ball. The planner would only have to make the sum of body velocity and the velocity added by the shoulder rotation come out right.

Allow the elbow to rotate, and you must add body velocity to the sum of the shoulder angular velocity times the shoulder-to-elbow distance, plus the elbow rotation angular velocity times the elbow-to-ball distance. And so forth for wrist and fingers.

But, since each axis of rotation is itself moving forward – with some velocity that is a sum of the higher-up rotations' velocities – during its own angular rotational motion, the calculation is nested. One expects to see the brain using a structured algorithm looking something like a nested tree with successive merges, finally comparing the score of this solution to your memories of previous throws. The calculation actually isn't limited to five rotational axes. The shoulder is notoriously mobile, moving relative to the backbone with the activity in the muscles of the neck, back, and chest. The hand too has a few minor axes of rotation. They all complicate the equation, easily moving you off one of the few good solutions onto one of the millions of worthless solutions lurking nearby. Furthermore, you don't just need one of these planners but quite a number, so many solutions can be tried in parallel. Each would be rated on an arbitrary scale of goodness, and the better-rated solutions varied to create a new generation of candidates – exactly what Darwin Machines are so good at.

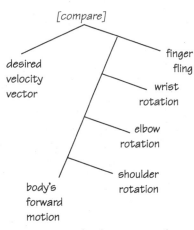

Segmented Throwing Plan
for an underarm throw at a novel target

THE PLAN IS ABSTRACT, NOT A LITTLE SIMULATION operating in real time. The resonances against which the judgements are made are pretty abstract, too. But the implementation gets less abstract and closer to an orchestrated set of movement commands. It's a bit like Chomsky's older idea of a deep structure and a surface structure, or the common mathematical technique for analyzing communications engineering problems: working in the frequency domain and later converting the results back into the time domain.

The throwing implementation is a different spatiotemporal pattern than that of the code that competes. Instead of the space being the few hundred minicolumns comprising the hexagon, the space is now a long list of muscles, each contracted or relaxed at various times in order to rotate the joints at the requested angular velocities. Temporarily you can imagine each minicolumn as connected to a muscle (though I'm sure that the truth is far more complex).

And, just as I suggested a little tune as an analogy to the spatiotemporal pattern of both the concept's code and the planner's code, I can also suggest a different analogy for the performance's spatiotemporal pattern: just imagine a fireworks display, one where an aerial bomb bursts into a shower, parallel curtainlike lines tracing downward in the sky (each analogous to the changes in the activity of a given muscle in the back-chest-neck group). But in one of the curtainlike descenders, another bomb bursts toward the right, showering activity changes into another muscle group (those that rotate the upper arm forward). Then (all while activity is continuing to change in all the prior groups) an elbow-rotating muscle group bursts into life, then a wrist, and finally a hand-finger group bursts into activity on the right side of the muscle list. So charting things this way, "muscle space" is left-to-right, and time is downward, and everything is happening at once, though the new things tend to drift to the right and lower down in the time chart. (We are plotting *changes* in muscle activity here; there's a background of firing in all muscles, from when you tighten up everything as you get set to launch). If the muscles are temporarily imagined as the keys on a piano, the music would be a densely packed arpeggio building into a precisely timed finale.

The most crucial events are those that happen late, during periods of high velocity movement; a little error there in timing, and the implementation mistakes are much greater than when everything was moving slowly earlier in the launch sequence. Fortunately, those crucial high velocity muscle changes don't have to be planned in real-time simulations; the planning machinery can look ahead in "virtual time," as well as backward at the candidate virtual launch so far.

Everything matters: the massive orchestration of all the relevant muscles must be judged as a whole. Does it hit one of the effective solutions (the ball is launched at the velocity that your depth perception judged to be correct for the bocce setting)? Or does it miss, merely because the activity of one muscle was altered at the wrong time?

It's much like how language's planner (all those little roles to be satisfied in argument structure) can look at how the utterance works as a whole and then turn the winning version into another one of those fireworks bursts of activity in a set of chest, tongue, and facial movements, each with its own set of physical constraints. The language planner can also look ahead to the completion of the utterance while adjusting the middle parts, just as the throwing planner presumably looks ahead to the crucial high-speed actions when adjusting the plan for the body and shoulder components.

INDEED, MIGHT THE BALLISTIC MOVEMENT PLANNER be able to do double duty, serving as the structured utterance planner when not too busy with throwing or hammering? Or might the planner machinery have been cloned (as visual field maps seem to have been)?

Study of the aphasics who have trouble with novel hand-arm movement sequences suggests that cortical space is shared between language and hand-arm. Ojemann's core areas where both auditory and oral-facial sequences are confused by cortical stimulation (mentioned back on page 65) also suggest shared function. The muscle groups used for the implementations of speech, throwing, and hammering may be different, but the segmented neural machinery of look-ahead-and-behind planning might be shared.

Throwing certainly has the equivalent of nested embedding: the launch sequence involving fingers is embedded in the environment created by wrist rotation, which is within the elbow's, the elbow's within the shoulder's, and all within the context of the slower body motion. (Derek, notice the "order of attachment" constraints here, perfect for the ordering of your obligatory roles!) So planning is naturally segmented in the manner of that earlier throwing planner diagram, which looks so similar to those diagrams of sentences like "I think I saw him leave to go home" with all their nesting.

Implementation in language has a series of constraints from conventions that have to be applied when converting the plan into the performance: word order or case markings, order of role attachments to the verb, and so forth. Throwing too has its local conventions, mostly from the length of your arms and the relative strength of your opposing muscles; converting a deep plan into the appropriate fireworks shower has to take all of these conventions into account. There aren't shared conventions for a whole community of throwers, but all throwers are constrained by the same Newtonian physics of launch and flight trajectories, learned in early life by calibrating body movements during play and by mimicking others.

If a Darwin Machine is used as the throwing planner, then there is another advantage: timing precision. That's extremely important during the higher velocity parts of the movements, the ones that cause the velocity to peak and fall off at the right time as the hand sweeps through an arc, and thereby launch the ball from the hand at the correct angle from the horizontal. (Speech has a similar set of high-velocity movements where timing is crucial – when timing is off, we say speech is slurred or foreign-sounding.) When the Darwinian throwing-planner competition produces a winner, it incorporates many losing hexagonal mosaics into the winning one, thus creating an even larger plainchant chorus, each hexagon of which is "singing" the winning "song."

The easy way to cut timing jitter in half is to increase the size of the chorus by a factor of four. (Doubling throwing distance while maintaining your success rate requires reducing jitter eight-fold, which takes a chorus 64 times larger.) A Darwin Machine might be able to shape up quality using a winning hexagonal mosaic of only a hundred hexagons but, if timing jitter matters, it may be advantageous to use much larger playing fields so that the winning mosaics are many times larger.

Ah, you may exclaim (as I once did): *that* must be the reason why hominid brain size increased fourfold in the last 2.5 million years – it's for throwing accuracy! Alas, a fourfold increase in mosaic size only buys you an insignificant 25 percent increase in throwing distance. (My general answer to why the brain enlarged is simply by analogy to economics: doing experiments is a lot easier in an expanding economy than in a zero-sum game, when you have to give something up in order to do the more-than-likely-to-fail experiment. And a hominid had to become a jack of all trades to survive the abrupt climate changes superimposed on the ice ages, which were too sudden for slow adaptations to help.) Size, about the only thing that can be measured about ancient brains, might have helped, but it can't be the main story.

THE ONLY PRACTICAL WAY TO GET MANY-FOLD INCREASES in hexagonal mosaics is to temporarily borrow cortical territory, much as the expert choir singing the *Hallelujah Chorus* borrows the inexpert audience.

As ever-larger hexagonal mosaics are created to reduce timing jitter in high-speed throwing, they may secondarily create coherent corticocortical connections. While one naturally thinks of large mosaics being created by expansion into contiguous territory, there is also (to be discussed in my next chapter) a way of borrowing distant cortex via coherent corticocortical connections (rather like singing along via a long-distance conference phone call).

The needs of throwing (where throwing twice as far or twice as fast is always significantly better for, literally, bringing home the bacon) may have driven the evolutionary changes in recruiting helpers, but other uses of the throwing planner might also benefit from them: language, planning for tomorrow, even music. And, if it's really a shared facility, improvements in anatomy for even better language performance could incidentally make throwing still better yet. (One isn't, of course, "throwing" words – if anything, one is throwing sentences.)

So don't make the mistake (as numerous people have done since 1981 when I first began discussing the role of accurate throwing in human evolution) of assuming that throwing is the *sole* driver of this common facility: *any* of the ballistic skills and higher intellectual functions could have driven its evolution. Some – say, throwing – might have been more important five million years ago, and others more important in the last several ice ages. But they all benefitted each other during the ascent of mind.

THE THROWING PLANNER has a number of useful characteristics, when viewed from the standpoint of what language needs. It can help shape up quality utterances, because it's already a Darwin Machine. It can provide planning space for nested embedding of phrases and clauses, because of its nested treelike features. It can help achieve timing precision during high-speed vocalization sequences, again thanks to the Darwin Machine's final product, the large hexagonal mosaic. And this oversized chorus might, in turn, have seeded "metastasises" in remote cortical areas via newly coherent corticocortical paths, cloning virgin territory.

But how might the structured Darwin Machine have interacted with the social calculus way of analyzing sentence structure, identifying arguments of the involved words? Very fruitfully, I suspect, because it can provide a segmented workspace that can house all of those phrases and clauses identified by argument structure. The progressive merging of throwing solutions seems a lot like the progressive merging of phrases and clauses that Derek emphasizes, where argument structure is mapped onto a tree. Training up a co-opted throwing planner into a sophisticated language planner using sharing-influenced argument tags might require a few additional refinements, but it looks like a good foundation – provided that the temporal lobe's nouns and their tags can readily participate in frontal lobe segmented planning.

DB: I think we have to be a little careful here in the analogy between executing a throw and building a sentence. The things that you regard as embedded in the throw – arm movements, wrist movements and the rest – differ from the phrases and clauses that are embedded in language in more than one way. First, an arm movement is not built up out of wrist movements, and a shoulder movement isn't built up out of arm movements: we're talking here about things which, while they share obvious commonalities, are simply different in kind from one another. However, every clause is a collection of phrases, one or more of which may be expanded into a clause, which in turn consists of a collection of phrases, one or more of which may be similarly expanded, and so on indefinitely. The same kinds of things are used over and over. Second, the number of units you use in a throw is finite and strictly limited – there are only so many body parts you can involve – whereas a sentence is potentially infinite, and certainly has no numerical limit.

WHC: Ah, but you are forgetting how arbitrary a hexagonal code is. It can be a movement, a word, a concept combination like "unicorn," a phrase, a clause, even a metaphor. It can represent nonsense, as in a mantra. (Ever hear the mantra that the Jewish Buddhists use to meditate? "Oy. Oy. Oy.") The neural machinery that links together modular movements doesn't know whether a code is ultimately a movement or a metaphor, it just structures what it is given in the way that a loom weaves yarn. A code for an analogy simply unpacks very differently than does a code for an entity or a state of affairs.

And a numerical limit might be a problem if the planning machinery is fixed in the manner of a railroad switching yard for boxcars (as I once diagramed ten years ago in *The Cerebral Symphony*, back before I knew the anatomical circuitry via which neocortex can implement a Darwinian process – that was *Calvin 2.0*, if we're going to keep track of versions). But rather than a fixed set of tracks and switches, I now think of it as more like a Lego or Erector set, one that allows you to build short squat bushes or tall spindly trees from the same set of building blocks. While there is perhaps some limit on the number of building blocks in the cerebral cortex, redundancy suggests that you could have tradeoffs, simply reducing redundancy (plainchant choir size) in order to have more independent branches (choral "parts," symphonic "voices").

The main thing suggesting limits is that "seven plus or minus two" human digit span, what makes it so hard to hang onto ten-digit phone numbers long enough to dial them, in comparison to seven-digit numbers. That limit might be the number of totally independent mosaics that can be managed simultaneously, without one dying out or several merging ("chunking").

There are also analogies to be made between trajectory planning and narrative projections, those blended spaces that Mark Turner talks about in *The Literary Mind*. Recall his example from the sailing magazine about a "race" between two boats whose journeys were actually 140 years apart:

> As we went to press, Rich Wilson and Bill Biewenga were barely maintaining a 4.5 day lead over the ghost of the clipper *Northern Light*, whose record run from San Francisco to Boston they're trying to beat. In 1853, the clipper made the journey in 76 days, 8 hours.

We deal easily with such metaphorical constructions, mapping the old journey onto our trajectory planning for the modern trip to create a "ghost" lagging behind. Perhaps that's because we have a lot of mental machinery for representing real trajectories and matching them up with memorized ones of the past, checking for "fit." Understanding one story by mapping it onto a more familiar story (that's what constitutes a parable) shows how we can operate mentally, once we have the structure for syntax and can use it again for even more abstract, beyond-the-sentence constructions.

This promotes "logic." One of the problems, of course, is that mapping can change the input space if you're not careful, contaminating your model of reality. Just remember what Dostoevsky said in *Letters from the Underworld*:

> But man has such a predilection for systems and abstract deductions that he is ready to distort the truth intentionally, he is ready to deny the evidence of his senses in order to justify his logic.

13

Corticocortical Coherence Promotes
A Many-Voiced Symphonic Sentence

My candidate for the augmented-protolanguage-to-fluent-syntax step can be stated succinctly (if densely) as: *the frequent use of Darwin Machines in the frontal lobe (mostly for ballistic movement planning) leads finally to the achievement of corticocortical coherence in the arcuate fasciculus and a spatiotemporal code common across the cortex, so that, in throwing-free moments, embedded phrases and clauses can be handled in other Darwin Machines at some cortical distance from the one for the symphonic sentence, fully assembled.*

A series of hundred-dollar words, if there ever was one. I actually, so help me, tried to explain this coherence concept over lunch to Ruth and Elihu Katz, the Israeli couple. I didn't succeed in persuading them why having a uniform-across-the-cortex code was so powerful. They have high standards for an explanation, and I think that I must have sounded like someone arguing that a common European currency like the Euro was so logical that a system of foreign exchange (frequent money changing each time you cross a border) was unlikely to exist. Alas, the inefficient often persists in the real world – we have to change money to go over to Lugano in the

> Why do I require an hour to give this lecture when all I have to say really could go into roughly six sentences? Because I could not utter six sentences which were not so heavily charged with ambiguity that no one in the end would get the picture that I am trying to formulate. Most human sentences are in fact aimed at getting rid of the ambiguity which you unfortunately left trailing in the last sentence.
> —JACOB BRONOWSKI, 1967

next valley to the west – which is one reason why I dislike relying on efficiency arguments. For every perfection-of-the-eye example, there are a dozen evolutionary examples of the equivalent of a bureaucracy stuck with an inefficient way of doing something because it can never back up and start all over again with an improved system.

Well, lunchtime was hardly an appropriate setting to explain the first eight chapters of *Cerebral Code.* I never got to the role of corticocortical coherence in nested embedding, which is where the common code really shines. It seems capable of making syntax an everyday, subconscious task. Now that we've discussed Darwin Machines, coherence, and throwing's segmented planner, it is easier to see how they all interact with the up-from-social-calculus argument structure.

The essential nature of the little role links can be seen if you try to imagine a *lingua ex machina* without them, merely using the segmented planner version of the Darwin Machine and parsing via boundary words (try hanging candidate phrases and clauses onto workspace trees, using simple rules such as taking the noun after a preposition and its modifiers and making a phrase out of them). Alas, you will be left with a lot of ambiguity (multiple candidate trees will remain), and not much way to resolve the empty subject and object categories of a sentence such as "John needs someone to work for." But adding role links allows ambiguity to be quickly resolved, at the lightning speeds of language comprehension and production.

THE DEEP STRUCTURE CONSTELLATION FOR PLANNING need not operate in serial-ordered real time, but it does need to be packed and unpacked in a speedy way, effortlessly handling never seen before combinations of words. You can see the need for this most easily when it comes to placeholders (words such as "that"; pronouns whose referents may be in preceding sentences). If necessary, you can expand on the placeholder, providing the full name or phrase.

This is part of what is called binding in linguistics, but the need for placeholders may have originated in the inherent limitations of working memory. We often speak of "chunking" when a particular string of words takes on an identity of its own. Most people can remember a string of about seven random digits, such as a phone number, for long enough to repeat it back (or dial the number). But they have trouble with longer strings – unless some of them form familiar chunks, such as the 1-212 string for New York or the 44-171 string for London. You also see short-form substitutes in acronyms (the way we write "VS" as a shortcut for "Villa Serbelloni") and internet addresses (the Rockefeller Foundation is rockfound.org). It's really seven *chunks* that you can easily handle, not seven digits or words. You may use the short form at a certain level of operation but you usually need to unpack it eventually. You must be able to query the workspace where the long form is kept.

I assume that something similar is true for a sentence's subsidiary phrases and clauses: that a short form will do for competitive purposes, so long as it can be related to the long form when the time finally arrives for the successful sentence to be "read out" into surface structure and speech. This suggests that messages can be sent back and forth between the Darwin Machine performing at the sentence level and the various Darwin Machines implementing the clauses and phrases. And that must require the coherence I discussed in chapter 8, so that a long-distance code could be formed up on the fly, even for seldom used prepositional phrases like "with one black shoe."

Assembling words into associations ("black shoe") can be easily done using superpositions of hexagons, the kind that you get near borders where one hexagonal mosaic (the *S* for "shoe") overlaps with another (*B* for "black"). Form up an *SB* mosaic and, at its edge, superimpose it upon the code for "with," and you have a prepositional phrase. Keep going and you might achieve a territory of clones, each of which contains the superimposed codes for the eight words of "the tall blond man with one black shoe." It's the Bickertonian utterance length problem in protolanguage, and Sontag's breakfast table advice about brevity when speaking to Italian waiters in English. There are simply too many words, and you don't know which modified what, so that you make "blond black man" errors.

Doing all the association via superpositions at a borderline between territories does get to be awkward – but there's another, better way. The coherent replica of a hexagonal mosaic in a distant cortex allows, say, eight codes to be superimposed with ease (it just takes eight corticocortical paths terminating in the same area). It would seem, at first glimpse, to produce an equally ambiguous superposition. But reciprocal corticocortical links allow you to have your cake and eat it too, as they support structuring. It's all like a fancier version of the *Hallelujah Chorus*.

THE BACK PROJECTION FROM AREA ALPHA TO AREA BETA (on, of course, a different one-way street) can use the same code, and that means that beta can contribute to maintaining a chorus above a critical size in alpha (they are, presumably, always adapting and thereby falling silent). It would be like missing choir practice but

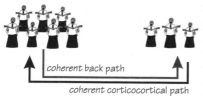

participating anyway via a conference phone call – and perhaps making the critical difference that keeps the performance from faltering.

Alpha's backprojected spatiotemporal pattern might not need to be fully featured, nor fully synchronized, to help out with beta's chorus. It might be like that sing along technique called "lining out," where a single voice prompts the next verse in a monotone and the chorus repeats it with melodic elaboration; some singing at a fifth or an octave above the others, some with a delay, and so forth.

The backpath could also include procedural prompts, just as choirmasters and folk singers manage to include exhortations with the desired text. Procedural prompts provide one way of resolving ambiguities when decomposing embedded phrases during production by, in effect, querying an audit trail. ("Who mentioned X? Sing it again, the whole thing!") With such structural links connecting the top-level hexagon's spatiotemporal pattern to subsidiary ones, there's no longer a danger that the mental model of the eight-word amalgamation "the tall blond man with one black shoe" will be scrambled into "the blond black man with one tall shoe."

The same mechanisms that clarify prepositional phrases probably help us to understand full sentences with independent clauses ("I think I saw him leave to go home"). The closed-class words,

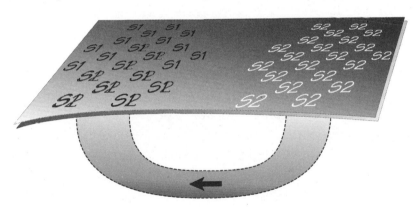

Coherent corticocortical paths can:

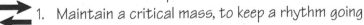 1. Maintain a critical mass, to keep a rhythm going

2. Superimpose one pattern on a distant one (S2 onto S1)

3. Disambiguate winning superpositions by reading out the contributors.

because they are limited in number, can probably all be handled as special cases, each with their own completion requirements regarding role links.

Verbs have more multifaceted completion requirements. Each verb has a characteristic set of links: some required, some optional, some prohibited. The conglomeration feels like a proper sentence only if all the obligatory links are satisfied and no words are left dangling, unsupported by a structural role. "Give" requires three nouns with appropriate role tags, "sleep" cannot tolerate more than a sleeper except via a prepositional phrase.

WHAT KEEPS THE TOP-LEVEL HEXAGON happy enough to reproduce effectively in a copying competition with other variant interpretations, such as that "blond black man"? Presumably, a few alternatives assemble in parallel until one gains the strong "legs" needed to allow it to become robust enough to establish hegemony. If, in "I think I saw him leave to go home," the "leave" link stumbles, the "saw" hexagons might not compete very effectively, and so the top level dangles.

So the "meaning of the sentence" is, in this model, an abstract cerebral code whose hexagons compete for territory with those suggesting alternative interpretations. Phrases and clauses require coherent corticocortical links to contributing territories, having their own competitions and tendencies to die out if not reinforced by backprojecting codes. Weblike crosstalk between subchoruses presumably occurs, and may be quite useful so long as it remains weak enough not to show up on the audit trail.

It starts to look like a choral work of many voices, each singing a different tune but with the requirement that it mesh well with all the others. Indeed, the symphonic metaphor might be appropriate for the more complex sentences that we can generate and understand. Certainly the reverse-order analogy to Benjamin Britten's *Young Person's Guide to the Orchestra*, the all-together version being succeeded by the various voices playing separately, is the best metaphor I know for the read-out process that converts the parallel-structured plan into serial-ordered speech.

THOUGH THE COMMON CODE FOR MANY CORTICAL AREAS is obviously a Good Trick, is it *the* Good Trick that transformed RA-augmented protolanguage into fluent syntax?

One quick qualifying test is to consider the implications of efficiently linking the concept filled temporal lobe with the prepare-for-action frontal lobe, with a common code replacing the degenerate codes – and then dropping back to the old system, with incoherent paths forcing a reliance on slowly established associative links. Does it degrade gracefully, as communications engineers try to achieve with digital packet-based systems?

Without coherence, you'd still have a vocabulary (the temporal lobe still works). You'd still be able to plan some nonlanguage actions (you'd pass many of the neuropsychological tests for frontal lobe functioning), but your ability to quickly invent new trial run associations would suffer. Not only couldn't you form up a syntactic sentence to speak (except for stock phrases), but you couldn't judge sentences that you heard someone else speak because you could no longer judge the quality of your trial interpretations, whether they were nonsense, good guesses, or sure things. Your quality associations would be too slow for the windows of opportunity, and the results would be of poor quality because not shaped up very far by Darwinian copying competitions in the brain. And so your performance on language tasks would drop back to something like protolanguage, a wide choice of words but with novel sentences limited to just a few words to avoid ambiguity.

Another type of pathology I can imagine (chapter 11 of *Cerebral Code* has many more) concerns the hegemony requirements of the top-level hexagonal competition (call it the alpha mosaic). Suppose that there have to be N_{action} hexagons singing in the plainchant chorus before an action sequence is triggered (or, in the comprehension version of the language task, you decide the problem is solved and you can move on). Suppose that, in order to communicate with subchorus beta, it takes only N_{link} singers in alpha. Now suppose there is noise in the backpath, raising the critical number needed in alpha in order to keep beta singing. What happens if N_{link} becomes larger than N_{action}? Well, you couldn't incorporate distant clauses and phrases – you could neither read them out nor have their maintenance affect the top-level competition in alpha. Only the *incoherent* version of the alpha code would arrive in beta and, unless it was the incoherent code for a common phrase that beta would recognize, it would be ineffective.

So degraded coherence might well cause most aspects of syntax to degrade even more abruptly. If you pull the incoherence card, it will read:

> Do not pass *syntax*,
> go directly to
> *protolanguage*.

COHERENCE, AS I BRIEFLY MENTIONED EARLIER, can also help concepts to establish colonies or branch offices in distant areas of cortex. To avoid the delays inherent in using concept resonances in distant places, you could import some of the more frequently used resonances into the frontal lobe. Nouns that started out as temporal lobe specialties could secondarily operate out of the frontal lobe, following such a metastasis.

In a two-level Hebbian memory system, the long-lasting resonances are usually produced by a sufficient number of repetitions of the spatiotemporal firing pattern. If beta's mosaic is frequently seeding a chorus in alpha, then a resonance for it might also develop in alpha (perhaps not within the projection area of the coherent bundle, but somewhere in the territory of the mosaic secondarily generated thereabouts). In computers, this would be known as a cache (keeping frequently used code as close as possible to the processor). But it need not be a temporary resonance (as the cache analogy suggests), as it could be consolidated there (which is why I used the colony and branch office as analogies).

Furthermore, it need not be just the code for concepts; it could be code for performance, the little subroutine that it takes to quickly perform certain algorithms (the so-called "cortical reflexes" so handy for quickly hitting the brakes if someone shouts "Stop!"). The only real difference between the arbitrary spatio-temporal code for a sensation and that for a movement is whether it meshes well with the output pathways from the cerebral cortex and actually moves muscles in a coordinated way.

Within much of the cortex, code is simply anonymous code. If a spatiotemporal pattern can be copied, it may serve as a code; if it can be coherently sent over long distances, it may become a code common to many neocortical areas; if it fits the requirements of output pathways, it may even find its way out of the brain into the real world.

OTHER HIGHER INTELLECTUAL FUNCTIONS (music, planning for tomorrow, logic, playing games with rules) may, more generally, benefit from the neural systems that are so essential for syntax. Any task that requires the progressive improvement of quality would benefit from syntax's Darwin Machine. The discovery of order amidst seeming disorder might become much easier. The segmented planner suggests a way of creating new levels of abstraction for relationships, a way to compare relationships and generate metaphors – while still being able to decompose the whole into specific actions, such as speaking a sentence. (Sometimes, we can't get the output aspect together –we "know things of which we cannot speak.")

Thought often has to span many possible levels of explanation and locate an appropriate one. As we try to speak usefully about a subject like language or the brain, we are often torn between dwelling on rock-solid details and speaking in terms of perhaps too abstract generalities. We need them all, but we can only speak about one at a time.

We duck when we see someone cock an arm to throw a stone at us because we are predicting: we recognize the beginning sequence of a small spatial story, imagine the rest, and respond. Narrative imagining is our fundamental form of predicting.

When we decide that it is perfectly reasonable to place our plum on the dictionary but not the dictionary on our plum, we are both predicting and evaluating. Evaluating the future of an act is evaluating the wisdom of the act. In this way, narrative imagining is also our fundamental form of evaluating.

When we hear something and want to see it, and walk to a new location in order to see it, we have made and executed a Plan. We have constructed a story taking us from the original situation to the desired situation and executed the story. The story is the plan. In this way, narrative imagining is our fundamental cognitive instrument for planning.

When a drop of water falls mysteriously from the ceiling and lands at our feet, we try to imagine a story that begins from the normal situation and ends with the mysterious situation. The story is the explanation. Narrative imagining is our fundamental cognitive instrument for explanation.

–MARK TURNER, The Literary Mind, 1996

DB: There's an interesting issue here about the relationship between immediate memory limitations and sentence structure. You mentioned the "need for placeholders" in conjunction with chunking. Remember that placeholders were also needed for quite another purpose: if you didn't have every obligatory thematic role of a verb represented by something, there were too many ambiguities for the hearer to process long and/or complex sentences. But immediate memory limitations may have played their part, too, in the following way.

It may be sheer coincidence, but the number of possible thematic roles is in the vicinity of seven. You have the three that are most often obligatory, AGENT, THEME, GOAL, then the optional ones, TIME, PLACE, BENEFICIARY, INSTRUMENT. (Some linguists will suggest more, such as SOURCE – "I bought it from Bill" – and maybe one or two extra, but nobody thinks it's much more than seven). Certainly you hardly ever, if ever, find a clause that contains more than seven thematic roles, by the broadest criteria – certainly not in spontaneous speech. Then looking down the hierarchy to the phrase level, you often find a phrase with more than seven words – you wouldn't need to be Holmes or Watson to find dozens in this book, I'd imagine – but I doubt you'd find one with more than seven units, sub-phrases, or clauses. And certainly none of these sub-units would be longer than seven words. In other words (no pun intended), you take words and chunk them into phrases, then each of these phrases into a bigger phrase or a clause, then the clauses into a sentence, and so on up the line. You will be handling words far in excess of immediate memory limitations, but at no level of the operation will the *chunks* you're working with add up to more than seven at a time, and most times you'll have a comfortable margin of two to four units.

None of this by itself accounts for the stunning automaticity of speech – never has so much speech been uttered by so many with so little thought. However, structured chunking does remove from speech what would otherwise be a serious brake upon it. It's a nice case of language killing the bird of ambiguity and the bird of memory limitation with one stone, so to speak.

WHC: Let me try to summarize some likely steps – perhaps "ramps" might be the better word – along the way to the linguists' Universal Grammar:

> ▷ Symbols, those abstract stand-ins for real things and categories like "nothing," are the first step. It's now clear that a number

of species can master such concepts with skillful teaching, even if only a few (like vervets) use them in the wild. And they rarely invent new ones.

▷ Small collections of symbols with a compound meaning, corresponding to the short sentences of protolanguage. Clearly a number of species are capable, with tutoring or rearing in a language-rich environment, to comprehend (and sometimes even produce) such brief sentences.

▷ Longer collections of symbols that would be hopelessly ambiguous without structuring clues. A standard word order buys you some clues, the little words of grammar buy you some more. Intensive language rearing might get this through to various species, substituting for the acquisitiveness and inventiveness that human children seem to come with, without giving them everything that most children possess by the age of three. (However, such an intermediate level of syntax has not been identified in either children or stroke patients.)

▷ The full-fledged grammar beloved of linguists, what self-organizes in childhood from listening to language or watching a fluent sign language. Functionally, this too might be attained by intensively rearing nonhuman species during critical periods of early life, but humans might remain unique in the effortless acquisition of all those things that add up to nested embedding, empty categories, movement, and so forth.

And for completeness, let me add:

▷ Literacy, the written version of language, requires extensive tutoring. Some individuals have brains that cannot master reading despite fully-fledged spoken language.

This makes advanced language acquisition something like predispositions for a disease: you can acquire lung cancer if you work hard enough, but the genes sure do change the chances of "success." You can have the predisposition without the disease, and vice versa.

There's no doubt but that human genes combined with human culture give the infant a big leg up on acquiring phonemes, then words, then protolanguage, then structuring long sentences and narratives. Some of the various up-ramps leading to advanced language abilities could be steeper than others, more dependent (as is our reading ability) on tutoring. But apes might have the circuitry without having such epigenetic aspects as acquisitiveness; we'll never know how much of advanced language they can master until we try hard to rear infant apes with lots of enrichment. Maybe syntax is for them the way reading is for us – or maybe their brains really do lack some hominid-only hardwired circuitry. Until we know better, it might be best to view Universal Grammar genes as affecting the predisposition to softwire in certain patterns via experience or invention, not via some innate hardwiring present at birth. And to remember that syntax, however acquired, makes possible all sorts of more abstract meanings:

> We typically conceive of concepts as packets of meaning. We give them labels: marriage, birth, death, force, electricity, time, tomorrow. Meanings seem localized and stable. But parable gives us a different view of meaning as arising from connections across more than one mental space. Meaning is not a deposit in a concept container. It is alive and active, dynamic and distributed, constructed for local purposes of knowing and acting. Meanings are not mental objects bounded in conceptual places but rather complex operations of projection, binding, linking, blending, and integration over multiple spaces.
>
> –MARK TURNER, *The Literary Mind*, 1996

14

The Pump and the Slingshot

The achievement of a coherent corticocortical pathway connecting independent Darwin Machines is, I think, one of the most important things that happened during the last five million years of hominid evolution. But it's surely not the only one. Faced with multiple causes (and any language-origins book will supply a plethora of interesting candidates, nearly all of them more congenial to the philosophical mind than "throwing words"), you can try to sort them out with fast-track considerations.

Given two candidates, both capable of getting here from there, one is likely to be faster. This doesn't mean that the other is pre-empted (they're not really *alternatives*); it can surely continue to play a modifying (and perhaps stabilizing) role as the faster one sprints along, both of them modifying brain structures as improved functions pay off. But the faster is likely to have caused

> There is no step more uplifting, more momentous in the history of mind design than the invention of language. When *Homo sapiens* became the beneficiary of this invention, the species stepped into a slingshot that has launched it far beyond all other earthly species in the power to look ahead and reflect.
> –DANIEL C. DENNETT, 1996

more profound alterations in the brain circuitry – and perhaps in brain size.

I especially like the Bickertonian scheme for evolving syntax from a nonlanguage foundation in the social calculus of reciprocal altruism. That's because altruism has such an extensive growth curve, and I'm always judging evolutionary advantages by their potential for *repeated* growth. So many evolutionary inventions are "one shots": once you invent a digging stick or a carrying bag, you can't just keep reinventing it for additional credit. You have to do something different for your next act. Even inventions with growth curves will often plateau: aquatic mammals, for example, find they can swim faster by reducing their body hair. This reduction can be repeated for further advantage, but there's a limit, as you can only become so naked. Most evolutionary Good Tricks do not have long growth curves.

A long growth curve is one of the nice features of accurate throwing: no matter where on the growth curve you currently are, throwing twice as far or twice as fast will improve the payoff still further (more high-calorie, low-toxicity meat is usually a dietary improvement). So one of the things that I like about cooperation is that it too, at whatever stage you're at, keeps being advantageous in so many circumstances. Doubling the size of the sharing group always has another payoff: eventually one could get such social organization as systematic sharing with the disadvantaged, a system of laws to minimize conflict, and chancy joint endeavors with an agreed upon sharing of any yields.

Being able to repeat the course for additional credit is an important consideration given that, in an evolutionary system where there are multiple plausible "causes," the fast track may be the important one, even if the slow ones might have also succeeded given enough time. There are many plausible candidates for what enlarged our brains, elaborated our social behaviors, and gave us structured language and thinking; the issue may come down to which was fastest – or which had the best "curb cut" potential for secondary uses.

FURTHERMORE, EXTENSIVE *ALTRUISM* is on the short list of major inventions since our last common ancestor with the chimps and bonobos, five million years ago – another major improvement that needs an evolutionary explanation. In my opinion, the big beyond-the-chimps developments are:

> *accurate throwing* (not just flinging) and its associated rehearsal,
> *extensive toolmaking* (especially tools to make tools),
> *reciprocal altruism* (the expansion of food sharing and such),
> *symbols* (not just species-specific calls but arbitrary on the fly inventions denoting shared meaning),
> *protolanguage* (real words used in short combinations),
> *structured language* (long sentences with recursive embedding of phrases and clauses),
> *planning* for uncertain futures (not just the seasons),
> *logical trains of inference* (that allow us to connect remote causes to present effects, and on to future implications),
> *ethics* (much of which requires an ability to estimate the consequences of a proposed course of action, and judge it from another's standpoint),
> *concealed ovulation* (the lack of obvious estrus behaviors tended to force males into prolonged sharing with a female and her offspring),
> *games* with made-up rules,
> *music* (not just rhythm but structure such as harmony),
> and our extensive offline *creativity* (an ability to speculate, to shape up quality by bootstrapping from rude beginnings, yet without necessarily acting in the real world).

The two major preadaptations we've been discussing, planning for accurate throwing and role categories for altruism and argument structure, both strike me as being good fast track candidates because they're capable of being re-used in a further round of improvements. I have no idea which was faster, but I think that it will prove useful to compare either of them to the many other candidates for what was important in hominid evolution that lack long growth curves.

Furthermore, both elaborated sharing and accurate throwing are likely to have been under strong selection during the ecosystem crashes that occurred every several thousand years during the ice ages when the climate abruptly cooled or warmed. These repeated events were *not* the ice sheets themselves, let me hasten to say. Rather, they were the fastest of the many types of climate instability that the planet has suffered in the last three million years or so.

Let me summarize briefly, using the introduction that I gave at Bellagio when doing my stint on the after-dinner circuit. Each resident usually gives a brief show-and-tell in the music room or upstairs in the conference room, some time during his or her month at the Villa Serbelloni, on some past or current project. Derek did syntax, so I did the "physics for poets" version of the abrupt climate change story that I wrote for *The Atlantic Monthly*.

EVER SINCE THE DAMMING UP of the original Panama Canal about three million years ago, when North and South America finally drifted together, the Earth's climate has been unstable. There had been a tropical path for the ocean currents between the Atlantic and Pacific Oceans but, with the rise of Panama, there's now a long loop of ocean currents between the North Atlantic and the southern oceans. Sometimes this loop (it's actually more like a conveyor belt, going north on top and going south near the ocean bottom) shifts into an alternate mode of operation, with drastic climate consequences.

The most vulnerable part of the current path is when it turns around in the North Atlantic Ocean, via diving from the surface to the ocean bottom in the whirlpools of the Greenland and Labrador Seas, and then heading south. When this turnaround shifts to occur well to the south of Iceland, things change elsewhere too. Our ancestors saw such an occasion as a catastrophic cooling, even if they lived in Africa rather than Europe. The cooling wasn't necessarily frigid, especially in the tropics – the new daytime temperatures were more like the nighttime temperatures before the shift, with the new nighttime temperatures shifting to proportionately cooler. The real problem with the climate change was how abrupt it was: just a matter of a decade or two.

Coolings like these are the equivalent of jacking up the landscape a thousand meters in elevation. Even the plants on the valley floors are unhappy, not only because of the cooler temperature extremes but because of less rainfall. Plant species growing up on the mountain sides would be suitable for the valley floors, but there isn't time for them to get there before lightning strikes set the dry forests ablaze. The landscape in many places must have soon looked like those pictures of Brazil and Southeast Asia we saw during the 1997-98 El Niño, where lightning and forest-clearing fires got out of control and burned vast areas. Familiar ways of making a living vanish, even in the tropics.

If this global cooling had taken 500 years to happen, it would have been difficult but not a catastrophe, as the mix of plants and animals would have gradually changed to emphasize the new climate conditions. Each generation could have made their living in the manner their parents taught them. But instead of ramping down to the new temperature, it stepped down (so say the isotopes and air bubbles in the ice cores from Greenland, which preserve a tree-ring-like series of layers from the last ice age). With major changes in just a few years, innovation was the only way to survive. Hominid populations must have crashed – and, in doing so, fragmented into many isolated groups.

AS THE POPULATION FRAGMENTED, some of the subpopulations turned out to possess a majority of what, beforehand, were minority traits. It was just the "luck of the draw." These days, we are surprised when the court clerk draws a jury with a majority of a minority group, given that the jury pool had only 20 percent of the minority group. Similarly, out of a jury pool with the usual 10 percent left-handers, you can sometimes randomly draw a jury, most of whom are left-handers. Some of the hominid sub-populations, just as improbably, found themselves with a majority of food sharers, or with an unusual number of individuals with a passion for throwing things.

For a few generations, the only plentiful food was likely grass. If you couldn't eat grass directly, there was a premium on being able to eat animals that predigested the grass for you. And some groups would also, by the luck of the draw, have had more altruistic tendencies than others. Those groups assembled by chance would have had, in such circumstances, an interesting advantage: they would have wasted a lot less time arguing over a food discovery and spent more time looking for additional ones after sharing it out. A better-fed group might survive the crash whereas the groups that fought constantly did not.

Though serious objections have been raised over the years to both hunting and reciprocal altruism scenarios in hominid evolution, the objections may not apply with any force during the abrupt decade-long population bottlenecks, simply because of the chance sorting and selective group survival that occurs in bottleneck times. Though some of the changes might be lost as selection pressures relax with the return of less transitional ecosystems, the abrupt disruption repeats a hundred generations later to surprise a culture that has forgotten the survival tricks of the previous episode. Still, some will possess the epigenetic traits that helped their ancestors to survive similar conditions: the tendencies to share, or to practice aimed throwing.

It all suggests an interesting scenario. Just imagine starting with chimpanzee-like tendencies to share meat and fling branches.

The dry season came early and the grazing animals were scrambling up hillsides and into improbable gullies in search of isolated patches of grass. *Hominids too had difficulty finding all kinds of food; they too were visiting improbable places and digging up roots to eat, especially for their water. After weeks without a good meal, those small to start with began to die, carried off by minor illnesses that they would have ordinarily survived.*

Droughts were nothing new, but this one persisted. It was cooler, too. The forests became quite dry and then, struck by lightning, they burned. Within a dozen years, the hominid population broke up into many fragmented groups; just by chance, some had a majority of individuals who tended to share food, even though they had been a disadvantaged minority in the original population. Those groups that fought over the remaining food finds wasted a lot of time and energy doing so; those who shared had more time to look for additional food, they suffered fewer injuries, and they survived better. Freeloading strangers from neighboring groups seldom took advantage of them because groups were few and far between.

Several years later, the grasses were doing well on the burned landscape. The grazing animals that survived the drought and the intensified hominid hunting found themselves in a boom time. Grass, grass, and even more grass. The hominids that had survived were scattered around the landscape in groups of only a few dozen, and mates had to be found locally because there weren't enough resources to eat in between adjacent groups, limiting visiting opportunities. They had survived not only because they fought less but because, again by chance, they had more children who were always throwing rocks at anything handy.

The easiest targets for the adult hunters were herds visiting waterholes. Because the animals packed tightly together as protection against the usual four-legged predators, they made an easy side-of-the-barn target – just fling a tree branch into the herd's midst, and some animal (it didn't matter which one) would be knocked off its feet and trampled by the fleeing herd. Those hunters who could club the hapless animal before it got back on its feet could provide a nice high-calorie meal for friends and relatives (it was, after all, too much meat to eat all by yourself).

Of course, tree branches were soon in short supply in the vicinity of waterholes, so rocks had to be lobbed instead. And some rock shapes were more effective than others at knocking a herd animal down temporarily. If a rock were thrown against another rock, sometimes it would break into the right shape. But even if it didn't, some rock fragments proved to have sharp edges, particularly handy for getting through the skin of the dead animal and carving off a leg at the joint.

Within a few hominid generations, the landscape looked less barren. The grass was succeeded by bushes and trees, and eventually by a mature ecosystem that was more suited for the new regime of rainfall and annual temperature extremes. Visiting between hominid groups became easier, and soon group size grew to be more like the old days. Food habits, too, drifted back toward old favorites, as many individuals were likely tired of such a heavy diet of meat. Soon food was plentiful enough so that one didn't have to share just to be eligible for a handout later from someone else's bonanza, so there was some drift back toward rugged individualism. In another ten generations, the stories of the bad years were lost to the cultural memory; the important things to the boomtime culture were very different from those in bottleneck times.

Many dozen generations later, another abrupt climate change occurred. Again the hominid population crashed within ten years, fragmenting into small groups —some of which had, by chance, the right genetic variants to emphasize food sharing and/or hunting ability. Having happened before, there were more of such variants around.

SUCH "RELAXATION" AFTER A SELECTION PRESSURE is lessened is a standard feature of evolutionary theory, but this one comes with a climate instability that repeats the stress, pumping it back up ever further, concentrating the already concentrated even more. This gets around the well-known weakness of group selection scenarios, that they backslide via cheaters – it's like a leaky tire, all right, but you can keep pumping to maintain a minimum level, thanks to repeated fragmentation and recovery. Furthermore, there is something of a ratchet that counteracts backsliding: meat is a prized food among the chimpanzees (and likely our common ancestor), and the social prestige of the successful hunter likely provided more reproduction via sexual selection.

Group selection happened, not because of groups competing like football teams but because most subpopulations starved, done in by the abrupt environmental change. Groups that had only average collections of traits likely perished. Only those groups lucky enough to wind up with "the right stuff" got through the terrible times.

Such fragmented bottlenecks, where lots of experiments occurred in parallel, likely happened many hundreds of times as brains grew larger. Any one episode only had to change things a little bit, because of this pump. Several dozen abrupt coolings have happened since our species, *Homo sapiens*, arrived on the scene, and they shocked people just like us: suddenly, the name of the game changed, and the way your parents taught you to make a living no longer sufficed, making it imperative to discover new ways within just a few years.

There wasn't much change in our brain size with the episodes during the most recent ice age, however, probably because something even more important had happened in the prior ice age that give our ancestors even better mental tools with which to get through the abrupt hard times: it was Dennett's slingshot. My guess is that structured thinking became much easier because of the coming together of the preadaptations, thanks to enough improvement in corticocortical coherence. We not only began to grow our culture with the aid of a truly versatile language, but we could use the same structured mental abilities to plan ahead and to reason more logically. Success at hunting and cooperation yielded the limelight to the higher intellectual functions that we so prize: syntax, planning, logic, games, and music. Together, they made possible that combination of foresight and altruism that we know as ethics.

For a glimpse of what happens to the higher intellectual functions without syntax, consider the case of Joseph, an 11-year-old deaf boy. Because he could not hear spoken language and had never been exposed to fluent sign language, Joseph did not have the opportunity to learn syntax during the critical years of early childhood. As Oliver Sacks described him:

> Joseph saw, distinguished, categorized, used; he had no
> problems with perceptual categorization or generalization, but
> he could not, it seemed, go much beyond this, hold abstract
> ideas in mind, reflect, play, plan. He seemed completely
> literal – unable to juggle images or hypotheses or possibilities,
> unable to enter an imaginative or figurative realm . . . . He
> seemed, like an animal, or an infant, to be stuck in the present,
> to be confined to literal and immediate perception, though
> made aware of this by a consciousness that no infant could
> have.

Perhaps that's what our ancestors were once like, back before the higher intellectual functions arose, sailing up out of some nonintellectual curb cut. Perhaps the appropriate metaphor isn't Dennett's slingshot but the curb cut, the skateboarder's substitute for a ski jump.

DB: Looks to me as if two of our pre-syntax candidates, carryover from reciprocal altruism's cognitive categories and ballistic movement's planning circuits, are compatible with slow language improvement over a few million years.

WHC: And "compatible" is probably the right word. Carryover seems possible, but that need not translate into full performance. It might have been too slow for many behavioral windows of opportunity, the carryover more useful for planning agendas than for social repartee. Fluency and capability are different matters. It might be like comparing the production of 13-year-olds with 3-year-olds.

DB: But your corticocortical coherence seems different to me. There's a real threshold there, a big transition from diverse cortical sites having to talk with one another via incoherent paths and slowly learned code translations. Once you can recruit enough temporary members for your sending choir, you can do on-the-fly associations between structural elements such as phrases and clauses housed in different bits of cortex.

That, it seems to me, would have made structured thought and talk far more fluent – and thus a capstone candidate for what triggered the flowering of art and technology seen late in hominid evolution, after brain size itself had stopped growing.

WHC: Yes, if you consider the reciprocal altruism and ballistic planning routes to be syntax-capable stones in an archway, then something like corticocortical coherence might be a capstone candidate, a development that really makes syntax stand on its own and fly.

If carnivory was indeed the catalyst for the evolution of sharing, it is hard to escape the conclusion that human morality is steeped in animal blood. When we give money to begging strangers, ship food to starving people, or vote for measures that benefit the poor, we follow impulses shaped since the time our ancestors began to cluster around meat possessors. At the center of the original circle, we find a prize hard to get but desired by many. . . this small, sympathetic circle grew steadily to encompass all of humanity – if not in practice then at least in principle . . . . Given the circle's proposed origin, it is profoundly ironic that its expansion should culminate in a plea for vegetarianism.

–Frans de Waal, 1996

The right to search for the truth implies also a duty. One must not conceal any part of what one has recognized to be true.

–Albert Einstein

15

Darwin and Chomsky Together at Last

For four decades, the study of our species and its unique capacities has been delayed and disrupted by a controversy that should never have come about. The evidence that all species, including our own, developed through natural selection operating on genetic variation is so overwhelming, one might think that only those driven by some ideological agenda could fail to accept it.

The evidence that language is an innate, species-specific, biological attribute that must possess a specialized neural infrastructure is so overwhelming, one might think that only those driven by some ideological agenda could fail to accept that, too.

It ought to have been obvious that a blending of the Chomskyan approach and the Darwinian approach could go a long way towards explaining what we are and resolving the apparent paradox that has hag-ridden the human sciences for centuries: that we were produced by the same forces as other species, yet behave so differently from other species.

This book, then, is an attempt to bring peace to a conflict that should never have broken out in the first place, and to show, contrary to so much that has been written over the past few decades, that the approaches pioneered by Darwin and Chomsky are fully reconcilable. Before summing up that attempt, it may be worth while to consider how the conflict came about.

IN DOING SO, WE HAVE TO BEAR IN MIND THAT SCIENCE is not the coldly objective, squeaky clean process it's sometimes portrayed as being.

It is a fallible process carried out by humans who, like all of us, are driven by passions and presuppositions that aren't always recognized for what they are. If we weren't ornery, cussed primates who wanted to be alpha animals, we wouldn't have the energy to drive good new ideas to the point of acceptance. If primates hadn't developed reciprocal altruism, we wouldn't form alliances to back up those good new ideas and do down the bad old ideas that stand in their path (and we wouldn't have language, so we wouldn't have any kind of science). And of course, in an alliance, you back your own guys against the other guys, come what may.

On top of all this, science has a history, and that history shapes the way in which issues are framed and helps determine the sides people take on those issues. It all began after the publication of *The Origin of Species*, when Darwin came into conflict with Max Muller, a leading linguist of his day. Taking on himself the mantle of Descartes, who had opined (philosophically filling out the Judeo-Christian framework) that humans and animals were irrevocably distinct, Muller declared language to be the Rubicon that "no brute will dare to cross." Darwin, on the other hand, declared in correspondence with Muller that one "fully convinced, as I am, that man is descended from some lower animal, is almost forced to believe a priori that articulate language has developed from inarticulate cries." In response, Muller derided what he termed Darwin's "bow-wow" and "pooh-pooh" theories of the origin of language, and his followers were successful in persuading the Linguistic Society of Paris to ban all presentations on language evolution from its meetings and publications.

The Paris ban is defensible in that it saved the world from a great deal of half-baked speculation. The better part of a century would elapse before people knew enough about language, human ancestry, and the brain to begin to make halfway intelligent guesses about how language might have evolved. The broader implications of the ban, however, were less fortunate. Lines had been drawn in the sand, and those lines would largely determine how linguists and evolutionists would interact for decades to come.

THE IRONY IS THAT DARWIN HIMSELF might not have been opposed to the idea that language was a kind of instinct. Throughout his life, he was moving from early sensationalism and Lamarckian thinking toward the idea of species-specific behaviors as the consequence of instincts that, in turn, had to have been derived (somehow) from natural selection.

But Darwin, strong at both ends of the intellectual spectrum – on empirical and comparative studies, and on overarching, metatheoretical conceptions – was always weaker on the middle ground, and especially on the mechanisms that would underpin the processes he so presciently described. Perhaps the most poignant image of scientific might-have-beens is Mendel's groundbreaking paper, which would have solved Darwin's deepest problems, moldering for sixteen years in his library, unread, its leaves not even cut.

If Darwin had read Mendel and incorporated Mendelian genetics into his theory, that theory and the physiological approach to mental breakdown spearheaded by Emil Kraepelin could have merged to form a true science of human behavior and avoided the wasteful detours into behaviorism, Freudian psychology, and cultural anthropology that were to mark the first half of the twentieth century. Instead, the evolutionary movement got sidetracked into eugenics, became marginalized, and remained peripheral to studies of human nature up to and beyond the mid-century. Throughout the behavioral sciences, it was as if Darwin had never been. And, to add insult to injury, the Nazis highjacked eugenics and made sure that, for decades to come, belief in innate characteristics would tar its holders with a neofascist brush. In the mid-century consensus, language formed part of culture, the human mind at birth was a tabula rasa, and cultural evolution had somehow projected our species out of the domain of biology altogether.

Ironically, the first serious blow against this consensus was struck not by some embattled evolutionary biologist or geneticist, but by a scholar who (the first of several poor P-R moves) chose to fight under the improbable banner of Descartes. Noam Chomsky's brilliant review of Skinner's *Verbal Behavior* exposed the weak intellectual underbelly of the consensus and opened a breach, into which attacks from a variety of disciplines soon began to pour. But, given his choice of Descartes as sponsor, Chomsky's approach looked, from the evolutionist trenches, less like an assault on general learning theory than a reaffirmation of human separateness. Quickly the debate veered back to those lines in the sand drawn by Darwin and Muller almost a century before.

These military metaphors should not be mistaken for some authorial attempt to jazz up the issues. For Chomsky, and for quite a few others on both sides, this was indeed war, a war to be fought with ideological fervor and with no quarter given or taken. Chomsky in particular perceived himself as an isolated fighter, lumping most positions other than his own into an empiricist-continuist Goliath against whom he could play righteous, stone-slinging David. His combination of an insistence on the biological nature of language with a refusal to look at the origins of that nature – and his blanket statements about the futility of any such enterprise – turned off many in the evolutionary community who might otherwise have been supportive. Others, more hard-nosed, responded in kind and denounced Chomsky as a spinner of absurd and irrelevant theories wholly devoid of empirical support. The lines in the sand became formidable entrenchments, behind one or other of which most workers in the behavioral sciences felt obliged to join up.

In the murky light of this all too real world of modern science, plain and obvious facts – like that Darwinism has to be right and Chomskyism has to be right – tend to look a whole lot less obvious than they otherwise would. Ignore all the warts of either one of them, focus on all the warts of the other, and anyone might conclude that one is right, the other wrong, and never the twain shall meet. Hopefully this book has shown why such a conclusion is misguided, and these last few pages have shown why, despite all this, so many have followed that misguided path.

PEACE COMES, OF COURSE, AT A PRICE. No right-minded person would expect that two separate lines of thought, conceived for totally different purposes and developed on totally different lines, would just dovetail neatly together, with no need for trimming and fitting. What we hope to show is that such trimming and fitting, while it might seem a threat to dearly held beliefs on both sides, does not in fact require either side to cede any significant territory. Let's just summarize the process and then see what, if anything, anyone has to give up.

What we have described is a perfectly legitimate evolutionary process, one that has time and again fashioned apparent novelties out of long-established organs and faculties. Reciprocal altruism, great-grandfather of so much we would want to preserve, started out as pure selfishness, with just a touch of foresight. If you scratch my back, I'll scratch yours – but if you let me scratch yours without returning the favor, I'll eventually dump you and find someone more accommodating. Keeping track of the interchanges, making sure you weren't giving much more than you were getting, became central to the social life of many primate species. And the only way one could avoid being short-changed was to set up abstract categories labeled "Giver", "Given", "Receiver" (or AGENT, THEME, GOAL in linguistic terminology) and store an event in memory in such a way that one could recover, automatically, the occupant of any given role.

Without some such way to structure events, our ancestors might have stumbled into protolanguage but could never have created true language. There may be symbols, but strings of symbols without structure quickly become too ambiguous for real time analysis and response.

AND THE SYMBOLS THEMSELVES? Darwinians may not even have to entirely jettison Darwin's belief that "articulate language developed from inarticulate cries." Although cries and words have too many differences – including even the acoustic wavebands they use – for a simple, straight-line continuist theory to work, a few elements of the original call system, linked with gestures, pointing, and other communicative tricks, might have played a part in the early forms of protolanguage.

Any evolutionary account of a new trait has to provide at least two things: a plausible selective pressure that would have served the trait, and a degree of inheritable genetic variation on which to work. With regard to the emergence of protolanguage, we have chosen a selective pressure from extractive foraging rather than the (recently more popular) social intelligence of primates. In the real world, food comes first, socializing second. And most theory-of-mind, Machiavellian-intelligence accounts extrapolate from modern chimp and bonobo societies rather than realistically reconstructing the hominid situation, which is subject to much more stringent environmental pressures than affect modern tropical apes. After all, the only animals other than ourselves to have anything that can transmit variable factual information, as language can, are bees, and bees, like our ancestors, are extractive foragers and use their language to help in their extractive foraging.

The requisite variability, in the earliest stage of protolanguage, would have involved the capacity to recruit one's fellows, by whatever combination of gesture and sound, to make particular foraging choices (led to a relatively unguarded carcass only a few hours old rather than to some decaying remains ringed by aggressive scavengers, for example). Thus not merely the power to communicate but some skill in handling the act would have been selected for at the same time, leading to increments in social intelligence as well as communicative ability.

Once protolanguage was established, the theme tagging from the social calculus could have been mapped onto it to immediately give structured utterances, but for one thing. To create a structured utterance requires that neural signals be transmitted over long distances within the brain, relayed through many points, and merged with or added to other signals without losing their coherence. If the brain's capacity to sustain a coherent message is limited, then it's a more reliable strategy to send out symbols for utterance one at a time, rather than first combining them into a single structured message. True, that limits you to very short utterances (four or five symbols maximum, preferably less) but why would you need more than that for exchanging information about food sources (or even a bit of basic gossip)?

Accordingly, the further development of language had to await two developments: increase in the number of available neurons and improved connections between the various parts of the brain involved in language. Protolanguage itself, in the beginning at least, probably didn't serve as a direct selective pressure toward increased brain size. Initially at least, such things aimed throwing and percussive hammering may have increased the number of "spare" neurons (that is, neurons that could be co-opted on occasion for linguistic purposes). Aimed throwing, because of its long growth curve (limited only by the power of human arm muscles), may have been particularly effective in this respect (there is no such thing as throwing too far or too accurately). But as time went by, protolanguage must have played an increasing role in brain growth. The people who believe a complicated social life caused language have the right steps in the wrong order. Language of any kind, however primitive, would have made social life enormously more complicated. Once lying and tale-bearing became possible, you had a lot more information to store and you had to be able to figure out how accurate it was if you weren't going to be perpetual patsy in your buddies' intrigues. Social life plus protolanguage was like a muscle-building machine for the brain. And above it all was the attraction of having as a mate someone who got words out (however few) quickly, clearly, and appropriately – as opposed to someone who coughed, hesitated, and said duh-duh-duh.

So you may be able to knock down a running rabbit at thirty yards. You may be able to con everyone in your group into believing what a nice guy or gal you are, while still managing to grab most of the goodies for yourself. But these are not things that leave any marks in the fossil record. That's why it was possible for hominid brains to balloon to modern human size without any of the new artifacts or new behavioral patterns that you'd expect high intelligence to yield. To create novelty demands a special type of thought, a very special type indeed.

WE DON'T HAVE SPACE HERE to get into the relations between language and thought, which have buffaloed philosophers for centuries. Suffice it to say that to change things, to do new things without a lot of groping around, you have first to plan them in your head. And to do that requires that you are able to maintain thoughts – which are simply patterns of neural impulses – in your brain over times long enough to let you assemble and reassemble them. That's exactly what you do when you're putting sentences together. That's why the Great Breakthrough didn't happen way back in the lower Paleolithic. It wasn't that we weren't smart enough, just that we weren't the right kind of smart.

So the creativity that most clearly marks us as human had to wait on the crossing of the same threshold that gave us our language. Given that *Homo erectus* and Neanderthals had big brains too, we can assume that they were traveling the same route. Did our own immediate ancestors get there first, was there really the clash between glib-tongued humans and tongue-tied Grisly Folk that fiction writers like Wells and Golding imagined? Or were the capabilities more even, with mere accidents of technology or political history giving our ancestors the edge? Hopefully, ongoing research into periods of human-Neanderthal co-existence, in both Europe and the Near East, will yield at least part of the answer.

We can be surer about what happened to our own folk. Even when signals could be maintained through the merging of two word representations, that wasn't much help. Single-merger capacity would give you just prefabricated utterances of two words. But you could produce those just as well in protolanguage, sending out words one at a time, with less risk of something going wrong. All signal coherence then gave you was a little more speed in delivery. It couldn't even give you a good argument structure mapping, because lots of verbs take more than one obligatory argument. And doubling your capacity to two merges wasn't much better, even though that meant a 100 percent improvement. But here a new accelerating factor began to come into play. The brain is a parallel, not a serial processor: it can do lots of things at the same time. So, assume you have capacity to sustain coherence through two merges. You simultaneously merge A with B and C with D. That counts as just one merge. Then you merge AB with CD.

With two merges you can assemble four-word messages. You could properly construct a single clause utterance like "Big men eat meat." But nothing any longer or more complex than that. And remember that the protolanguage machine could produce strings of four or five words – without any structural constraint, granted – before multiplying ambiguities caused the process to grind to a halt. So there's still no decisive edge for a language machine over a protolanguage machine. But then a mere 50 percent increment in what coherence buys – from two to three merges – doubled your potential from four to eight-word utterances. Now for the first time, multiclause sentences and multiclause thoughts come within your grasp. A piddling 33 percent further increase would again double the potential length of sentences to as many as sixteen words.

By this time, the Baldwinian processes would have come into effect; our ancestors would have been elaborating means to make sentences more parsable. The best of these would have been reinforced by neural adaptations, and natural selection would have been winnowing the resultant variation to yield something like the "no argument without a non-argument" principle and the empty-category algorithm, both described in the appendix. Again, female mate selection would have driven the process and selected systematically for more efficient language processing. And so we arrived at a language that, apart from having different words, would show no significant differences from the kinds of language we speak today.

NOW IT'S TIME TO ADD UP THE SCORE. What, if anything, has anybody had to give up? On the evolutionist side, nothing of any value. The processes we have here hypothesized as taking part in the evolution of language – exaptation, female selection, Baldwinian evolution, and so on – are all recognized processes accepted by a large majority of those working in the field of biological evolution. One might argue about the effects of particular processes at particular stages, but no principle has been violated, no macromutations or Lamarckian heresies have been smuggled in. Some of the more naïve forms of "call-system to language" might have to be junked, but that's no loss, since none has ever been worked out enough to merit debate.

What about nativists? Again, nothing of significance is lost. We have shown that no simple-minded continuist scenario and no amount of general-purpose learning will suffice to account for the emergence of language. If it did, big-brained hominids would surely have given us today's language a million years ago or more. We have shown language to be innate, species-specific, and supported by task-dedicated circuits – even if parts of those circuits may do double or treble duty in other tasks. We have removed language's origins from the shroud of mystery in which generativists preferred that it remain hidden, just in case some empiricist came up with a good story. Decades of stimulation mapping in the brain has shown that strictly locationist models of language – one module, one function – won't fly in the real world. But then it was Fodorian psychology rather than linguistics that promoted encapsulated modules. Most linguists didn't care enough to get as specific as that. And the model of language our approach entails is one toward which Chomsky's minimalism has been heading for a decade now.

On the plus side, let's suggest, for each of the two parties, one problem that our approach promises to solve. The problem for evolutionists concerns brain size; the problem for linguists concerns language acquisition.

WHY DID THE BRAIN CEASE TO EXPAND – even, if some figures for Neanderthals are representative, contract a little – when our species came upon the scene? After all, if evolution has been selecting for larger brains for millions of years, why not go on? If a brain of 1400 cc is good, why isn't one of 2800 cc twice as good? If our brains had really swollen as general intelligence machines, that argument would surely apply.

The obvious answer is, of course, that purely physical constraints apply: some say, "the human birth canal simply won't allow for bigger brains to be born." But that argument would have applied equally well when human ancestors had brains in the 400-600 cc range; if it didn't apply then, why should it apply now? The birth canal must simply have widened as heads swelled. In any case, even if we have hit some developmental wall, the argument still wouldn't apply. First, some humans have

WHC: It's not even clear that brain size is important for *anything* — except perhaps paleoanthropology, as sheer size is almost the only thing you can measure about ancient hominid brains. We just suspect that bigger is better.

brains 50 percent above the norm, so canal size couldn't stop a 50 percent increase. Second, even if it did, there's nothing to stop a development in which a still longer and larger development of the brain occurs outside the uterus. If the goal is viable, evolution can find a way.

A much better explanation is that the brain stopped growing because it was now big enough to end-run the biological version of evolution. Suppose, however shocking it may sound, that our computational tools, our modes of reasoning, are in fact no different from those of chimpanzees and that our only superiority lies in our higher level of neural message coherence, which allows us to build chimpanzee-level thoughts into impressive edifices (and doubtless have quite a few thoughts that are well beyond the reach of chimpanzees, too). Now, without novel reasoning devices, there is not much point in being able to construct longer trains of thought than we can now construct. The main limit on these seems to be the size of working memory, and working memory too might expand (and brain size with it) if, for instance, we came into contact with an alien species roughly equal to ourselves in computational power. Without that, or something like it, there's no selective pressure on working memory to expand. It nicely holds about the number of elements we can compute over; it's not obvious what advantage would accrue from increasing that number. And evolution has never seen the need to replace a Good Trick with a Better Trick, if the Good Trick works well enough and there's no competition. It's just not in the cards.

LET'S LOOK NOW AT A PROBLEM FOR LINGUISTS: the pace of syntactic acquisition. Typically, children acquire their first words around twelve to fifteen months, proceed in a couple of months or so from one-word to two-word utterances, and may thereafter remain stuck in the two-word stage for as long as six months before bursting out into what some acquisitionists have called "the syntactic spurt," which carries them, often in a matter of only weeks, to a stage in which they can produce a wide variety of biclausal sentence types. This herky-jerky trajectory has long puzzled acquisitionists, who, noting that children in the two-word stage can typically comprehend sentences far more sophisticated in structure than any they can produce, have talked about some mysterious "production bottleneck" that curtails their utterances.

First let's dispose of the production-comprehension asymmetry. This exists not because children have syntax they can't express, but because comprehension draws on a wider range of possibilities than production does. In comprehension you can use the syntactic structure or you can use pragmatics, semantics, context, plus anything else you can lay your hands on – direction of eye-gaze, to name just one – in order to figure out the message. In production, if you can't use syntactic structure, you've had it. So production is the only reliable guide to how much syntax children have and when they get it.

NOW LET'S TAKE THE OLD RECAPITULATIONIST IDEA and re-run it. Of course there is no general law that ontogeny recapitulates phylogeny – but it does sometimes, if there are good reasons why it should. A baby's brain is like the brain of a prelinguistic hominid or an ape, in that there are no words in it. The words have to be put there, one by one, in the first instance. Now if it is correct that all our neocortical neurons are there at birth, then a baby has large enough neural choirs to sing out those words loud and clear. But there are two prerequisites for syntax: choirs and connections. The first couple of years of life are a time of dewiring and rewiring, as the environment works on the hand that nature dealt the child. On top of that, there's myelinization, essential if signals are going to be sent rapidly and frequently.

So until connections adequate to support complex messages are established, the child does indeed – has to – operate in protolanguage mode, dispatching words to the organs of speech one at a time. This does not stop the child from picking up some grammatical regularities such word order, and even some grammatical morphology, in languages that have such. How could a child help but do so, where virtually all words come with inflections or casemarkers attached? In all probability (because segmenting is a hard job), word-plus-morpheme combinations are acquired holistically. But as soon as adequate connections begin to get established, the picture changes rapidly. The onset may be as early as eighteen months or as late as three years, even in normals – but regardless of age, and at around twenty-five months on average, a torrent of structured language bursts forth. It was there all the time, potentially, just waiting to be let loose.

That torrent flows along the causeway already laid down by word-order regularities, but what comes out is not always grammatical in terms of the language of the local environment. To produce locally grammatical output, the child has to acquire the morphophonemic shapes and the functional properties of all the grammatical morphemes in the target language. The child does not, *pace* Chomsky, "determine from the data of performance the underlying system of rules" of that language. In the first place, as Chomsky himself would probably nowadays agree, there are no rules to learn. Rules are post hoc artefacts extracted by grammarians that might have some usefulness in helping adults with a full Piagetian deck to learn a foreign language. The child simply slots newly acquired grammatical morphemes into the overall schema that the brain, built as we have described it, provides. You might think that it would be harder to learn an item's functional properties than its morphophonemic shape – after all, the latter is just picking up and imitating a string of sounds. Wrong. Children seldom make mistakes with things like articles or prepositions or inflections (as long as the latter are regular, naturally), but it takes them sometimes till six or older to get the past tense forms of all the English irregular verbs.

So that's why language acquisition follows the course it does: a slow and hesitant beginning, a sudden spurt that takes one pretty close to adult competence in a few weeks or months, followed by a gradual filling-in of the picture that takes years. Pretty much the same course, as we have hypothesized, that language took when it first evolved, and for exactly the same reasons.

SO THE LONG-AWAITED MARRIAGE OF DARWIN AND CHOMSKY should be greeted with songs of praise on both sides. Like a lot of marriages that both families feared and fiercely resisted, it could well turn out a lot better than either hoped. Now at last the Montagues and Capulets of the contemporary human sciences can quit feuding and get down to some serious collaboration.

But on what, exactly? We can only say what we think needs doing, what we would like to do ourselves, or to see done by others.

Obviously our model of the Language Machine needs its tires kicked and some heavy test driving over the rougher patches. That's fine. Hopefully the overall design will stand up even if some of the parts need remodeling. Linguists, who are very good at this sort of thing, are sure to come up with all sorts of exotic linguistic phenomena that they will claim our machine couldn't possibly produce. We'll have to show either that it could, or that the phenomena can be reliably attributed to extralinguistic causes.

Then there's brain imaging and the other approaches to language physiology. We need more and better studies (PET scans, fast MRI, whatever the state of the art permits) of how the brain handles language on-line. Two things limit what we can learn from present studies. First, very few if any of them have focused on what happens when speakers produce completely novel sentences (by that, I simply mean sentences that the researcher doesn't know in advance and that the subjects haven't rehearsed before utterance – "Say the first thing that comes into your head" would be a good protocol). Second, most studies limit themselves to adult speakers using their native language. We need comparable studies of children and people speaking something other than their native language. If suitably noninvasive procedures can be applied to small children, we would like to see on-line scans of language production by children in the 18 to 30 months range, preferably the same tests repeated at monthly or bi-monthly intervals. We would also welcome comparative scans of language production by adult speakers in both their native language and a language they are just starting to learn, or an early stage pidgin, if they happen to know one.

THEN THERE ARE THE VARIOUS APHASIAS AND DYSPHASIAS. I just wish some experts in the field would get together and compose the Defective Speech Anthology (DSA). The DSA would consist simply of raw samples of speech by all the different brands of aphasics and dysphasics, with several samples for each condition. The most superficial reading on, say, Broca's aphasia, is enough to show that a very wide range of syntactic impairment is collected under that label. For each subject we'd need a full description, type and precise extent of trauma, age now and at onset, and so forth.

A colossal task, sure. So why take it on? Because the vast bulk of work in this area is, very naturally, from a clinical perspective, and therefore of limited use to anyone trying to find out how language is instantiated in the brain. But we now know enough about language to be able to determine the linguistic nature of defects rather precisely, and one hypothesis would be that if two individuals show an identical defect, even if they have been diagnosed under different syndromes, the same thing has gone wrong for them somehow. Of course that couldn't be the whole story. Maybe they would turn out to have things wrong with them in addition to what caused the linguistic deficit. Maybe two different conditions would (among other consequences) affect the same part of the brain in the same way. Maybe damage or loss in two different places could cause identical deficits. We don't know. But until we look at the evidence from this new perspective, we're not likely to find out. At worst, we'd find out a lot more about how the brain works.

One goal is a complete wiring diagram for the Language Machine. Although we've suggested how that machine was built and how it functions in a rather general way, we have not yet been able to provide a blow-by-blow account of what happens when you utter a sentence, like "X goes to A where it is joined by Y, and then X and Y represented by XY go to B, while at the same time . . ." in which X and Y are signals representing particular words and A and B are different places in the brain (and of course there would be the time in milliseconds for each move). Again, in attempting to piece together such a diagram, it would be amazing if there weren't many surprises that would force modification of the model in presently unforeseeable ways.

THEN WHAT ABOUT THE GENES? A lot of nonsense has been talked, pro and con, about "genes for language." It would be truly amazing if there turned out to be specific genes that do language and nothing but language. The genetic defect studied by Myrna Gopnik that seems to affect grammatical morphology is the best candidate so far, but its precise effects are still controversial and in any case it affects only a small part of the language faculty. The probability is that a number of genes indirectly conspire to yield language; hopefully, study of the dysphasias will help out here, for of course research is synergistic, and results from most of the areas touched on here ought to shed light on other areas.

Looking back now, into prehistory, we'd obviously like to see a richer record of our past. There could be surprises there too. If complex artifacts two million years old started turning up, it would be back to the drawing board with a vengeance. What seems more likely is a filling out of the existing fossil record. The really interesting additions to our knowledge may come from a better understanding of paleoclimatology and paleoecology, which may help us, far more than a handful of stone tools, to reconstruct the behavior of our remote ancestors.

More far-reaching consequences may come from a more informed exploration of the relationship between language and mind. In the early days of generative grammar, it was sometimes suggested that the study of language would yield profound insight into the workings of the mind. But this line was quickly dropped. Strategically, in the warfare described in the opening paragraphs of this chapter, it looked a better bet to claim that syntax, in particular, was totally different in its principles and mode of operation from anything else in the mind. Now that the war's over, we can take a second look. It could well turn out that our minds are no different from the minds of other primates – except that we, thanks to our large numbers of neurons and sophisticated connections, can keep a coherent signal going longer than they can.

But we must never forget that the whole point of research is to explore the unknown without too many preconceptions. So perhaps our deepest wish is that our work will lead in directions we never even thought of, to discoveries beyond the span of our imaginations. If our model leads to things of that caliber, it will matter little whether the model itself lives or dies. Better by far to open doors on the unknown than to lock them with dogma.

Acknowledgments

We wish to thank the Rockefeller Foundation for hosting us for a month at their Bellagio Study and Conference Center at the Villa Serbelloni. We also benefitted from workshops organized by the La Jolla Origins of Humans group (sponsored by the Preuss Foundation and the Mathers Foundation) and the Center for Human Evolution at the Foundation for the Future. We got a lot of useful questions and advice from Yvonne Bickerton, Katherine Graubard, Ruth and Elihu Katz, and the other temporary residents of Bellagio; Jess Tauber, Peter "Throwing Words" Rockas, Elizabeth F. Loftus, Beatrice Bruteau, Blanche Graubard, Dan Downs, Chris Westbury, David Schoppik, Bart de Boer, Francis Steen, Gerhard Luhn, Heidi Lyn, Robert Berwick, Steven Pinker, Michael Rutter, and countless anonymous reviewers. We also thank John Sunsten, Stewart Brand, William Hopkins, Terry Deacon, Frans de Waal, Richard Dawkins, and Greg Ransome for helping us chase down illustrations and citations.

Linguistics Appendix

I n this appendix I shall try to show that the core phenomena explained by a Chomskyan universal grammar can be derived directly from the exaptation of a social calculus, plus a theta-role hierarchy, the Baldwin effects of the exaptation, and a procedure for joining meaningful units. The stakes are quite high. If I fail in this attempt, then a substantial part of this book must be dead wrong. If I succeed, then the account of language evolution given in this book is strongly confirmed.

An enterprise of this nature is novel as well as risky. People who have tried to account for the evolution of language have paid little if any attention to the details of

> Derek has aimed this appendix at readers accustomed to the linguistics literature and its conventions (like *iff* for "if and only if"). But even I can understand it.
> –WHC

syntactic analysis; people who have studied syntax in any depth have paid little if any attention to the exigencies of evolution. It is time to abolish this dual imbalance. Syntax certainly evolved, and evolution, equally certainly, determined what the properties of syntax should be.

Recently, Noam Chomsky observed that "a problem for the biological sciences that is already far from trivial" is "how can a system such as human language arise in the mind/brain, or for that matter, in the organic world, in which one seems not to find systems with anything like the basic properties of human language?" Chomsky goes on to remark[1] that "biology and the brain sciences . . . as currently understood, do not provide any basis for what appear to be fairly well-established conclusions about language." The purpose of this book is, of course, to accept this challenge and try to provide just such a basis.

However, what has to be done may encounter initial resistance among some syntacticians who have rejected any attempt to determine syntactic theory that includes evidence from areas other than synchronic syntax.[2] Such resistance is natural, even laudable, considering the nature of some attempts made by specialists in other fields, with little or no understanding of generative theory, to explain how language came to be. However, one should bear in mind a very early remark by Chomsky[3], that "theory is underdetermined by data" and that, consequently, constraints that go beyond the empirical ones may be required to decide between competing theories.

Such constraints are usually regarded as purely theory-internal, involving considerations of economy, elegance, consistency, and the like. However, I think that (with all due caution) a case can be made for using evolutionary considerations as a further constraint. Most of us agree that syntax evolved somehow, and it would be strange indeed if the process of its evolution had no bearing on its current state. Granted that the process described in preceding chapters is only one of a number of possible scenarios (even if a good deal more specific than most), it should be at least interesting to see the extent to which that process can be shown to determine the nature of syntax. But of course any such enterprise must submit to one essential restriction: what is proposed must take a form fully compatible with the "well-established conclusions" to which Chomsky refers in the passage cited above.

The Present Approach and the Minimalist Program

WHAT IS PROPOSED HERE has some obvious affinities with Chomsky's Minimalist Program.[4] However, one must point out a significant difference that is an inevitable consequence of the way in which the two approaches developed.

An ongoing problem for generative grammar has been its ongoing nature. The theory has evolved, over the past forty years, much as anything else evolves: that is, by throwing up, at each stage, a number of varying possibilities, and allowing the environment (in the form of a body of highly critical scholars) to determine which should live and which should die. The choice in turn determines the population of the next generation, reformulating and on occasion reprioritizing the problems assumed to be crucial to the overall enterprise. While there can be little doubt that this process, as a whole, has yielded ever fitter (that is, better fitting) theories, it does have a down side. At each stage of development, the theory contains elements inherited from previous stages that it doesn't really need (theoretical equivalents of the human appendix, so to speak) and that may be at variance with the spirit, if not the letter, of the current stage. The presence of these elements may in turn require adjustments that, in the long run, prove detrimental to the program as a whole. Some specific examples will appear later.

In the present approach, this problem is avoided by stating in advance the mechanisms that the theory will be allowed to incorporate, as well as certain mechanisms that will be disallowed on principle. For instance, while movement to both A- and A-bar positions is allowed, other forms of movement, such as those involving Larsonian shells[5] and Pollockian expansions of IP structures,[6] are barred. In the first place, both these strategies evolved as responses to problems involving serial order, and the solutions chosen were such as would preserve prior assumptions. Larsonian shells were motivated by the failure of c-command to account for a variety of structures,[7] and were calculated to preserve the validity of c-command by generating structures that would exhibit the "proper" c-command relationships. Yet c-command is not an empirical fact but itself a theoretical proposal, albeit a venerable one;[8] moreover, it cannot be deduced from any deeper principle, but must be stipulated. Clearly then, if it is possible to account for c-command phenomena by a mechanism that can be deduced, rather than stipulated, and that is independently motivated, the entire rationale for Larsonian shells disappears.

A second reason lies in the operation "Merge" which though it has become central in minimalist thinking, was absent from its earlier stages.[9] Once Merge, or something like it, is adopted, then the necessity for assuming the independent existence of tree structures into which lexical items are inserted simply disappears. There emerges instead the possibility of explaining puzzling phenomena on the basis of this attachment process, rather than by manipulating the prefabricated tree structures so as to move lexical items into configurations that never appear in surface structures. Chomsky himself appears well aware that this is the direction in which theory should move: as he remarked in a recent interview, "You will always do Merge if you can get away with it; you only do overt movement if there's no other way for the derivation to converge."[10]

A final reason for rejecting Larsonian and Pollockian solutions may carry less force with syntacticians, although I think it is equally legitimate. While there are good grounds for supposing that both A- and A-bar movements are neurologically real (in that both the extraction- and landing-site positions for such movements, as well as the movements themselves, must be tracked by the brain in the process of creating and comprehending sentences), the conceptual necessity of the positions and movements involved in Larsonian shells and Pollockian trees is much less well founded. While we cannot rule out the possibility that the brain does in fact go through all of the gyrations required by these as it creates and understands sentences, the assumption that it does not, that it does things in a more parsimonious manner, should surely be tested before resorting to more complex solutions.

The present framework, a sort of minimal minimalism, is extremely restrictive and limits itself to the following four mechanisms, plus procedures deductively derivable from these or resulting directly from their interaction:

A. Argument structure (the obligatory representation, dependent on verb-class, of one, two, or three arguments).

B. Obligatory attachment of all arguments to non-arguments.

C. A process of binary attachment of constituents, subject to compatibility between the features of the constituent attached and its immediately prior or immediately subsequent attachment.[11]

D. A hierarchy of thematic roles that determines their order of attachment to the right and left of the verb.

A few remarks on each of these mechanisms may be helpful here.

A IS ARGUMENT STRUCTURE, a mechanism that derives directly from the exaptation of the social calculus described in previous chapters. It results in the creation of what will be termed "Argument Domains." An argument domain resembles what has been described as a Complete Functional Complex;[12] it may be formally defined as follows:

1) *An argument domain consists of a verb and all the arguments of that verb, optional or obligatory, including obligatory arguments that are themselves argument domains.*

It follows from (1) that argument domains may be divided into two classes, minimal and maximal domains:

2) *The minimal domain of x is the smallest argument domain that contains x.*

3) *The maximal domain of x is the minimal domain of x plus any argument domain of which that minimal domain is an obligatory argument or part of such an argument.*

Consider the following examples:

4a) John loves Mary.
b) John told Mary that he knew Bill.
c) John told Mary that he knew that Bill had left.
d) John knows the man that he criticized.
e) John slept late because he forgot to wind his alarm-clock.

In (4a), the whole sentence is both the minimal and maximal domain of "John" and "Mary." The same applies in (4b, c), because in (4b) the subordinate clause is an obligatory argument of "tell" and in (4c) the most deeply embedded clause is an obligatory argument of "know," whose argument domain is in turn an obligatory argument of "tell." In (4b) the minimal domain of "Bill" is the subordinate clause and in (4c), the most deeply embedded clause, but in both cases its maximal domain is the full sentence, because each clause is an obligatory argument of the next highest clause. However, both (4d) and (4e) contain clauses that are not obligatory arguments of the matrix verb. Consider (5):

5a) John knows Bill.

b) John knows that today is Friday.

c) *John knows Bill that today is Friday.

As (5b) shows, "know" can take a clause as one of its two obligatory arguments, but as (5a) shows, it can also take a noun-phrase, and as (5c) shows, it cannot take both. (4d) is analogous in structure to (5a): the fact that "man" has a complement clause attached to it has nothing to do with the argument requirements of "know." This must be the case even though it is assumed here that the Vergnaud/Kayne analysis of relative clauses is correct[13], in other words that "the man" originates to the right of "criticized" in (4d). Thus in (4d), both the minimal and maximal domains of "he" are the embedded (relative) clause, while the maximal and minimal domains of "John" are still the entire sentence. In (4e), however, the minimal and maximal domains of "John" are simply "John slept late", because the rest of the sentence consists of an adjunct (not an argument of "slept"). The minimal domain of "alarm-clock" is the nonfinite clause "to wind his alarm-clock", and its maximal domain "because he forgot to wind his alarm-clock."

The above domain categories have obvious implications for such things as movement and binding, which will be dealt with at greater length in subsequent sections. As a first approximation, constituents may not be moved outside of their maximal domains, and, if bound, are bound in their minimal domains.

B IS OBLIGATORY ATTACHMENT, a mechanism that requires that every argument must be attached to a non-argument. A non-argument can be either of the two -N classes (Verb and Preposition) or any case-marker or other affix indicating, for example, topicality or thematic role (the present framework contains no principled distinction between bound and free morphemes). Consider (6):

6) Columbus discovered America.

Here there are two arguments ("America" and "Columbus") licensed respectively by the verb "discover" and a [+finite] INFL (in this case, the Past marking of "discover"). If we remove both licensing features in (6) (the verbal nature of "discover" and the finiteness of INFL) as for instance happens when we convert (6) into a noun phrase, the two arguments must be licensed by other means:

7) Columbus's discovery of America.

Now "Columbus" requires a genitive suffix to fulfill (B), and "America" requires a preposition. Note that these necessities are purely formal; there is no semantic impediment to understanding:

8) Mary considered that Columbus discovery America had done more harm than good.

Now consider what is known as "Exceptional Case-Marking,"[14] as in (9):

9) Mary expected Columbus to discover America.

Here, INFL is [–finite] and cannot license the attachment of "Columbus." However, because the verb "expect" is not required here to license another argument, it licences "Columbus" even though there is no verb-argument relationship between the two ("Columbus" remains an argument of "discover").

Note that because nothing stipulates that only one non-argument should be attached to each argument, there is no contradiction (in languages as diverse as Latin, Japanese, and Tagalog) in having all arguments licensed by their own affix, even those that (in English, Chinese or creole languages) would be licensed solely by verb or INFL. In other words, doubly or triply licensed arguments are not counter-examples to (B), because (B) states only a minimal condition.

Reference to creole languages brings up the point that these languages, which result from extremely unnatural forms of language contact where morphology is reduced to a minimum, still obey (B) without exception. Even where all appropriate grammatical morphemes have been lost, arguments not licensed by verb or INFL are still licensed by some non-argument; most commonly, lexical verbs are recruited to discharge non-argument functions, giving rise to the so-called "serial verb constructions" that are a common feature of creole languages. Thus in Sranan we find sentences like (10):

> 10) Mi teki nefi koti brede
> I take knife cut bread

to render "I cut bread with a knife", or like (11):

> 11) Mi teki buki gi en
> I take book give him

to render "I gave the book to him" (in Sranan, an English-based creole, there are no reflexes of E. "to" or "with"). The fact that Sranan and other creoles, emerging in a single generation from protolanguage-like pidgins in which constituents can appear randomly without any kind of licensing, immediately instal (B) in the absence of positive evidence is a clear indication that (B), although it may have originally arisen as an opportunistic strategy to assist parsing, now forms part of the human genome.

Thus (B) ties what has traditionally been referred to as "government" to the process of human evolution.

C, BINARY ATTACHMENT, is perhaps the single most important mechanism in the present framework, because order of attachment turns out to be crucial in matters of binding, coreference, and scope. For some time, binary branching[15] has been generally assumed as the most restrictive hypothesis; it forms, of course, the basis for the Merge process which is central to the Minimalist Program. The term "attachment" is used here because it seems to more accurately describe the process. Chomsky himself[16] has pointed out that the product of "Merge" could potentially be labeled as the intersection of α and β, the union of α and β, or one or the other of α, β; he concludes that the third possibility is the correct one. However, the term "Merge" is more appropriate for either of the first two processes; in fact, either α is attached to β, and the product is β, or β is attached to α, and the product is α (that is, modifiers are attached to heads, rather than vice versa).

Another difference between Attach and Merge lies in the actual node labeling. In the source just cited, Chomsky labels the product of a merged noun ("book") and determiner ("the") as "the" (equivalent to DP in other frameworks) rather than "book" (equivalent to NP). Indeed, since the work of Abney,[17] the DP assumption has been fairly standard. However, the main motivation for Abney's proposal was identical to that of Larsonian shells and Pollockian trees: that is, to create additional spaces for constituents to be moved to. This in turn reflects the long-standing and seldom questioned assumption in generative grammar discussed above: that there exist abstract tree structures and that lexical items are attached to terminal nodes in those structures.

This assumption, although not yet banished by the Minimalist Program, is now unnecessary. Trees are simply built from the bottom up by successive binary attachment, and because there is no X-bar theory[18], there are no constraints on the number or type of attachments beyond those imposed by the features in the lexical entries of the items to be attached. Movement is simply reattachment of an item at a higher level (see below for details of, and constraints on, this process); no prearranged "landing site" is required. Thus the immediate motivations for Abney's proposal no longer exist. For instance, the fact that in some languages possessive NPs and determiners can co-occur no longer requires that space be made for them. The solution lies in the lexicon. Lexical items may be specified with respect to whether or not they are phrase-final attachments — that is, whether attachment of such an item prevents further attachments to its phrase. In English, determiners are so specified, but not in all languages. Another of Abney's problems, gerundive NPs, likewise disappears once requirements of X-bar theory no longer need to be met.

However, Merge and Attach are similar in that both require feature matching or checking in some form or other. In attachment, the requirements of targets (heads or projections of heads) and the feature specifications of the units to be attached to targets must correspond (other constraints on the process are supplied by (D), the hierarchy of thematic roles, to be dealt with in the following section). Consider, for example, the attachment of final arguments (equivalent to "external arguments" or "subjects" in other frameworks; see next section for a detailed treatment of prior and final attachments) to nonfinite domains. This attachment is subject to the condition that the immediately prior attachment be one of Tense. If Tense is not present, the requirement of (B) for the final argument to attach to a nonargument cannot be satisfied. It can, however, be satisfied if the next attachment is to a non-argument that has not already been (and will not be, in any subsequent attachment) needed to fulfil another argument's (B)-requirement. Consider the following examples:

12a) Mary wanted John to leave.
b) *Mary wanted desperately John to leave.
c) Mary wanted desperately for John to leave.
d) *Mary persuaded Bill John to leave.
(Compare "Mary persuaded Bill that John should/had to leave.")

In (12a) "wanted," a nonargument which has not saturated its capacity to fulfil (B), is attached to the node immediately dominating the previous attachment "John"; "John" requires a nonargument, "wanted" supplies it, and the attachment is licit. In (12b), on the other hand, "desperately" must attach to "John to leave," and "desperately," an adverb, does not fall within the definition of non-argument given above; accordingly, attachment cannot proceed and the derivation fails. Again, in (12c), a permissible non-argument, the preposition "for", attaches to the node immediately dominating "John", licensing attachment. However, if as in (12d) another argument, "Bill", intervenes between a potential nonargument ("persuaded") and "John", the nonargument requirement of "Bill" saturates "persuaded" and an overt final attachment to the nonfinite domain is barred.

Argument Structure and Syntax

LET US TURN NOW TO D, the question of how thematic roles and the arguments that carry them get mapped onto a hierarchical structure, an issue that must be central to any theory seeking to demonstrate the evolution of syntax from argument structure. The process of attachment is crucially involved here; here, and indeed in all that follows, a guiding strategy will be to derive as much of the theory as possible from this process. Attachment, of its nature, is a serial, cumulative process, and the moves that compose it must follow a definite order. Here and elsewhere, the idea that order of attachment might play a significant role will be developed; in particular, it will be convenient to refer to attachment in terms of priority and finality, with respect to argument domains in general and minimal domains in particular. Thus attachment of X will be prior to attachment of Y *iff* X is attached to the tree before Y is attached. The attachment of X will be final *iff* X is the last argument of the verb of a given domain to be attached to that domain.

For reasons of space and simplicity, detailed discussion will be limited to English-specific mapping. We start with verbs that have only one obligatory argument. In English (and perhaps generally) the final attachment must be an obligatory argument. Accordingly, that argument (whether THEME, EXPERIENCER, or some other category is immaterial) must attach to an otherwise completed domain (in the case of English, to the left of that domain). If there are two arguments, one is oftenAGENT; in the unmarked case, AGENT forms the final attachment and THEME is attached directly to the verb, that is, prior to all other argument attachments.[19] If one argument is EXPERIENCER and the other is THEME,[20] the ordering depends on whether the verb is lexically marked as [+causative]:

> 13a) Bill fears ghosts.
> b) Ghosts frighten Bill.

(13b) can be paraphrased as "Ghosts cause Bill to be afraid"; the THEME argument thus acquires causative (agentive) properties and is treated syntactically as if it indeed had the role of AGENT. In (13a), however, the verb will not take a causative meaning, so THEME reverts to its normal (right of the verb) attachment.

Where there is a third (usually GOAL) argument, this attaches directly to the right of the verb, prior to the THEME argument, which now attaches directly to the right of the verb-GOAL complex. Note that if this order is reversed, the GOAL argument requires a preposition:

> 14a) Bill gave Mary a book.
> b) Bill gave a book to Mary.
> 15a) Mary bought Bill a present.

b) Mary bought a present for Bill.[21]

This leads us directly to the question of how alternatives to the unmarked ordering discussed above are handled. Consider passives:

16a) Mary was given a book by Bill.

b) A book was given to Mary by Bill/by Bill to Mary.

c) *A book was given Mary by Bill.

(16c) is usually explained by the inability of a participle such as "given" to assign Case (thereby forcing movement of "a book") although in (16a) and (17):

17) Bill has given Mary a book.

no problem arises. But this does not account for the contrast between (i) and (ii) in footnote 17, repeated here for convenience:

18a) Politics worries John.

b) John worries about politics.

Either we must assume two lexical entries for the verb "worry," with different subcategorization frames, or a more general process is at work.

The distribution of arguments noted above would follow automatically if there were a hierarchy of thematic roles in which positions in the hierarchy corresponded to positions in the ranking of prior and final attachments. In the latter, as we shall see, final attachments take precedence over all prior attachments, while prior attachments take precedence over subsequent attachments (excluding final attachments, naturally). This would suggest a thematic hierarchy of AGENT/Causer > GOAL > THEME/EXPERIENCER,[22] yielding AGENT/Causer as a final attachment, and GOAL as a first attachment prior to THEME. (There appear to be no cases of verbs taking AGENT, GOAL, and EXPERIENCER as obligatory arguments.) Any variation in the positions determined by the hierarchy would then be signaled by movement of a lower argument to a higher position (lower in terms of priority/finality, that is) and the demotion of higher elements to prepositional phrases.[23] In other words, if GOAL is promoted to final attachment (as in [16a]), THEME moves into its vacated position while AGENT must be demoted to a PP, while if THEME is promoted (as in [16b]), both AGENT and GOAL must be demoted to PPs.

Traditionally, movements such as those described above (A-movements) have been regarded as leaving gaps (empty categories, or ECs), as well as coindexed traces at the extraction site. There was always, however, something of a double standard involved. Objects moved and left gaps and traces (even though their position might still be case-marked and governed, as [16a] suggests) but subjects moved without leaving either a gap or a trace. Moreover, no one suggested that, in pairs like (18a,b), the object of (18a) moved to the subject position in (18b), leaving a gap ("John worries EC about politics"). Because A-movement involves for the most part[24] a reshuffling of positions, with predictable consequences, it will be assumed here that (in contrast with A-bar movement) it leaves neither a gap nor a trace.

So far, optional arguments have not been mentioned. These, in English, are attached to the right of obligatory arguments, in no particular order (as [16b] shows, there are no ordering restrictions even on obligatory arguments once these have been demoted to prepositional phrases). The position of optional arguments in the order of attachment between what have been traditionally described as "internal arguments" and the "external" one is logical in terms of priority and finality; both internal arguments are prior to all optional arguments and (by finality) the exterior argument is also superior to them. (We shall see, in subsequent sections, how final and prior attachments command and control nonfinal, nonprior ones.)

Arguments, whether optional or obligatory, can of course themselves constitute argument domains without limit, in any position. If an argument is complex (a complex phrase or another domain) it is assembled completely, along the lines described, before being attached to the main structure.

With regard to linear ordering, this is assumed to follow directly from the hierarchical structuring of constituents. If Merge is purely hierarchical, and requires a subsequent ordering in the phonological component (as some treatments suppose),[25] Attach is a concrete operation that specifies, for each attachment, the direction of attachment. It is therefore possible to take any syntactic tree and read off its terminal nodes, starting from the highest left-hand node and finishing with the furthest right-hand node; this gives the appropriate linear order.

Movement

THE MODEL PRESENTED HERE ASSUMES, in accordance with a long-standing generative tradition that still continues,[26] a model of movement consisting of three operations: (a) the insertion of the to-be-moved constituent in its "expected" position (the position dictated by the mapping procedures described in the previous section); (b) the copying of the constituent at the site to which it is to be moved; (c) the deletion of the original insertion.

Parsing considerations suggest that in any viable language, constraints would have to be imposed upon movement, otherwise anything could turn up anywhere, and the search for antecedents would become too costly in terms of time and energy to permit the kind of rapid, automatic processing on which language relies. In general, movement causes constituents to appear as postfinal (in English, extreme left-hand) attachments to argument domains; that is to say, once a final argument has been attached, an argument already attached within the domain in question may be copied and attached in postfinal position. However, attachment for copies of nonfinal WH arguments cannot be made directly to the attachment node of the final argument,[27] but requires the presence of a tensed auxiliary verb; attachment for copies of final arguments (as in [20], below) lacks this requirement, because deletion of the original constituent allows the copy to attach to nonargument INFL.

19a) John saw who?
  b) *Who did John see who?
  c) Who did John see?
20a) Who saw John?
  b) *Who who saw John?
  c) Who saw John?
21a) John thought that Bill said that Mary saw who?
  b) *Who did John think that Bill said that Mary saw who?
  c) Who did John think that Bill said that Mary saw?

22a) I know [Mary saw the boy].

b) *I know the boy Mary saw the boy.

c) I know the boy Mary saw.

As indicated by (19)-(21), movement can be to the left margin of a minimal domain (19-20) or a maximal domain (21). In (22), it might be objected that "the boy" and "the boy Mary saw" cannot be copies, since their reference is distinct. However, their reference is not distinct at the time the constituent is copied. The string (23) –

23) [the boy Mary saw the boy]

– exists before attachment to "I know" (that is, before the stage represented by [22b]) and at this stage there are simply two copies of "the boy"; the argument "the boy Mary saw" does not exist until after attachment and after the deletion of the copied constituent. At the stage represented by (23), the string could just as easily become a complete sentence:

24) The boy, Mary saw (him) [but not the girl].

As has been known since the 1960s, there are a number of restrictions on the extent of movement. For example, movement cannot occur out of the following constituents, even when the sentences would be fully grammatical without movement (in each case, movement is supposed to have originated at EC):

Relative clauses:

25a) *Who did you meet someone that knew EC?

b) I met someone that knew Bill.

Complex NPs:

26a) *What did John deny the rumor that Mary liked EC?

b) John denied the rumor that Mary liked tofu with broccoli.

Co-ordinate Ss:

27a) *What did Bill write letters and Mary played EC?

b) Bill wrote letters and Mary played the piano.

Finite adjunct clauses:

28a) *Who was Mary worried because John disliked EC?

b) Mary was worried because John disliked Bill.

Movement to the left margin of the matrix domain is impossible in all these cases because in none of them is the full sentence a maximal domain. In each, the minimal domain of the EC is its maximal domain. In (25), "someone that knew EC/Bill" is an argument, but not a minimal domain; the minimal domain is "EC that knew EC/Bill," where the first EC is the extraction site for "someone." Similarly in (26a), "the rumor that Mary liked EC" is an argument, but not a minimal domain; the minimal domain is "Mary liked EC." In (27), there are clearly two minimal domains linked by a conjunction, and in (28) the minimal domain of the EC is not an argument of "worried." In other words, movement is only possible within maximal domains – and, as (29) shows, not always then.

29a) *What did you wonder who John gave EC to EC?

  b) I wonder who John gave my address to.

Here, the embedded sentence is an argument of the matrix verb but its postfinal attachment position is already filled by "who." Postfinal attachment of an argument copy (or anything else) to a minimal domain "closes" that domain, making it inaccessible to further extractions.

    However, sentences such as the following, which seems to allow exit from a closed domain, are frequently cited in the literature?[28]

30a) What did you wonder how EC to plan EC EC?

  b) *How did you wonder what EC to plan EC EC?

Examples like this are supposed to demonstrate that a complement can move across an adjunct but an adjunct can't move across a complement (the second EC in (30a) represents the extraction site of "what," while the second is supposed to represent the extraction site of "how"; the first EC is of course PRO, coindexed with "you"). However, there is good reason to suppose that (30) has been misanalyzed:

31a) *What did you wonder EC to plan how?

  b) You wondered how to plan what?

  c) *You wondered to plan what how?

  d) *I wondered (that) to plan the party as a surprise.

(31a) shows that with "how" in situ (i.e. no crossing at all) the sentence is worse than (30a). The contrast between the two "surprise" questions (31b,c) shows that the reason uniting all three ungrammatical cases is that "wonder" requires a WH-word (or "if") as complementizer. If "how" is a complementizer, it is not a argument extracted from its minimal domain, therefore not an obstacle to the movement of "what" to the beginning of the sentence.

A further environment where movement is barred is that of sentential subjects. Although it has long been a goal of generative grammar to subsume all barriers to movement under a single mechanism, it remains an empirical question whether or not this is possible or even desirable. Its desirability may look obvious, but the relative parsimony of grammars should be judged not on whether they provide a single explanation for what has been traditionally regarded as a single phenomenon, but on which grammar requires the fewest principles and the least stipulation. In (32), the extraction site clearly lies within an argument of the matrix verb:

32a) *What did that John ate EC upset Mary?
   b) That John ate garlic upset Mary.

However, accounts of movement do not often note that

33) *Who did that John ate garlic upset EC.

or

34a) *What did that John could read Homer imply he knew EC?
   b) That John could read Homer implied that he knew Greek.

are just as bad as (32), even though (35) is fine:

35) What did John's reading (of) Homer imply that he knew EC?

Thus (32) does not represent an asymmetry between extraction from subject and extraction from complement, but rather a condition on attachment. The lexical specification of interrogative "do" must include the proviso that it cannot attach unless it can access, by (D), a terminal node representing an argument attachment. However, in (32)-(34), the only terminal node accessible to "do" is the one where "that," a nonargument, is attached. Note that in (35), (D) allows the auxiliary to access the node where "John," an argument of the domain "John's reading (of) Homer," is attached.

Another environment in which movement is apparently blocked involves the so-called "that"-trace effect:

36a) Who do you think EC left?
   b) *Who do you think that EC left?
   c) Who do you think Bill left EC?
   d) Who do you think that Bill left EC?

An enormous literature has been written about this effect, and many proposals have been advanced to account for it, most of them trying in some way to subsume the effect under some independently existing barrier to movement. However, a number of languages fail to show the effect. Indeed, sentences may be ungrammatical without the complementizer:

> 37a) Quien piensas que se fue? (Spanish)
>   "Who do you think that left?"
> b) *Quien piensas se fue?
> 38a) A who yu tink se a tiif di moni? (Guyanese Creole)
>   "EMPH who do you think that is stealing the money?"
> b) *A hu yu tink a tiif di moni?

Several writers have drawn attention to these problems[29] and attributed them to differences in the properties of the relevant morphemes in the different languages. In terms of the present framework, some factive complementizers require that the attachment immediately prior to their own have phonetic content, while others do not; it is worth noting here that Spanish "que," in contrast to "that," will also introduce nonfinites with null subjects:

> 39a) Tenemos que salir en seguida.
>   "We have to go out right now."
> b) *Tenemos salir en seguida.

It would seem therefore that barriers to movement arise from two distinct causes, attachment conditions and membership of minimal domains that either do not form arguments of maximal domains or have been closed by postfinal attachment. Though the conditions are disjoint, they are certainly no more complex than any other proposal for constraining movement. They have the further advantage that they invoke no more than the basic conditions of attachment and domain formation that underlie so many other aspects of the present account.

Determining Reference of Empty Categories

MOVEMENT HAS, AS AN INCIDENTAL CONSEQUENCE, the creation of a large number of empty categories. At the same time, certain A-positions may be forced to remain unfilled because there is no available non-argument they can attach to. However, all empty categories have to receive reference from somewhere (with the exception of "generic" complements such as those in [40] and cases of indefinite reference such as that in [41]):

(40) He ate EC and drank EC excessively.

(41) It isn't easy EC to get there from here.

Because empty categories are featureless and lack independent reference, and because part of the evidence for assigning reference to nonreferential constituents consists of matching their features with those of potential antecedents (we know, for instance, that "he" requires a masculine, singular, human antecedent), how do hearers determine the reference of empty categories?

In fact, there is a simple procedure, based largely on the order-of-attachment features "prior" and "final," which enables hearers to automatically determine the reference of empty categories, even where two or more empty categories occur within the same sentence. This procedure begins by determining whether the sentence contains A-bar constituents. If there is more than one such constituent, it takes the most deeply embedded constituent and determines whether there is a nonfinally attached EC. If there is, the A-bar constituent identifies with it; if not, it seeks an EC finally attached to a tensed clause. If there is one, it identifies with that; if not, it seeks an EC that lacks a prior attachment outside its minimal domain and identifies with that. The process is repeated (if necessary) until all A-bar constituents have been identified. Any ECs that have not yet been identified are then identified with an immediately prior attachment outside their minimal domain, if there is such an attachment, otherwise with the first final attachment outside their minimal domain. Any remaining ECs should receive a generic or indefinite interpretation.

The process can be illustrated by the following examples:

42) Who did Bill ask Sally EC to tell Mary EC to call EC?

In (42) the only A-bar constituent is "who." The first two ECs are final attachments to untensed clauses, but the third is a nonfinal attachment; therefore "who" is identified with it. The other two ECs both have immediately prior attachments outside their minimal domains: because "EC to call EC" is attached to "tell Mary" after the attachment of "Mary" to "tell," and because "EC to tell Mary EC to call EC" is attached to "ask Sally" immediately after the attachment of "Sally" to "ask," "Mary" and "Sally" respectively are the immediate prior attachments (and accordingly, the antecedents) of the second and first ECs.

> 43) Who do you think EC wanted EC to see Bill?

Again, "who" is the only A-bar constituent. Here there is no nonfinal EC, and of the two ECs, only the first is in a tensed domain, so "who" is identified with the first EC. The second EC has no immediately prior attachment, because "EC to see Bill" is attached directly to "wanted." The first final attachment outside the second EC's minimal domain is the first EC (a nearer antecedent than "you," the only other possibility) so "who" and both ECs co-refer.

> 44) Who did the boy Bill saw EC persuade EC EC to find someone EC to work for EC.

Here there are three constituents in A-bar positions, "who," "the boy," and "someone" ("The boy Bill saw EC" is, of course, in an A-position with respect to the matrix clause, but with respect to the minimal domain "Bill saw EC", "the boy" is in an A-bar position; similar considerations apply to "someone.")

We begin with "someone", the most deeply embedded, and find within its minimal domain a nonfinal EC (the fifth and last) with which it identifies. Similarly, "the boy" identifies with the first EC, also nonfinal. This leaves three ECs, of which one, that which follows "persuade", is nonfinal. Accordingly, "who" identifies with it. The same EC is attached to "persuade" prior to the attachment of "EC to find someone," so the two ECs share reference with "who." Finally consider the fourth EC, "subject" of "work for."

"Someone," the nearest potential antecedent, cannot corefer with it, because "someone" is a postfinal, rather than a final or prior, attachment to the EC's minimal domain. Accordingly, the fourth EC identifies with the third EC, the first final attachment outside its domain.

> 45a) Who did you expect EC to ask Mary EC to see EC?
> (Compare "I expected to ask Mary to see Bill.")
> b) Who did you expect EC to ask Mary EC to stay?
> (Compare "I expected Bill to ask Mary to stay.")

On the surface, (45a, b) differ by only a single word; however, the pattern of identification of the ECs differs sharply. In (45a), "who" again identifies with the third, nonfinal EC. In (45a). however, "stay," in contrast with "see," has only one argument, so that there is no nonfinal EC – and for that matter, no final EC in a tensed domain. "Who" must therefore identify with one of the untensed final ECs; because the second EC has a prior attachment "Mary" to identify with (in both sentences), "who" in (45b) identifies with the first EC. However, the first EC in (45a) identifies with "you," the first final attachment outside its domain.

Binding, Scope, and C-command

TREATMENT OF THE AREAS COVERED SO FAR has been unavoidably brief, omitting many nontrivial issues and leaving others without adequate discussion. In a single appendix to a single volume, it is obviously impossible to do justice to the wealth of both empirical data and theoretical argumentation that have emerged during the last four decades in the study of syntax. However, in order to show what the present framework is capable of, it seems desirable to take a single area and explore it in somewhat greater depth.

The area involving binding and scope is one that has been central to syntactic theory over at least the last two decades. Around binding theory in particular, a vast and controversial literature has accumulated, in part because of extensive cross-linguistic variation.[30] A variety of solutions have been proposed, and most treatments have found themselves obliged, at one stage or another, to handle phenomena within the same general area in rather different ways. However, the present framework is able to handle the entire area in a unitary manner; moreover, the mechanisms required to handle it are not (unlike other approaches) crafted specifically to fit the area involved. All that is required to handle problems of scope and binding is contained in notions that already form an inescapable part of the theory: those same notions of priority and finality of attachment that we have already seen at work in other areas of the grammar.

In its classic form,[31] binding theory describes the conditions that identify constituents without independent reference – pronouns and anaphors (reflexives, reciprocals, and the like) – by assigning mutually exclusive domains to these two classes.

> 46a) John washed himself/*him (where "him" = "John").
>
> b) John asked Bill to forgive him/*himself (where "himself" = "John").

But not all languages have both pronouns and anaphors: for instance, in at least one dialect of Haitian,[32] there is only one non-independently referential item in the third-person singular:

> 47) Li we li dan laglas la.
> "He saw himself/him in the mirror."

Languages with just two classes, pronoun and anaphor, tend to adopt an English-type distribution, with anaphors referring within their minimal domain, pronouns outside it. But there exist languages such as Greek or Icelandic with more than two classes. For instance Greek has an item "o idhios," literally "the same," which occurs within the maximal domain of its antecedent but, unlike the reflexive form "ton eafton tou," does not have that antecedent within its minimal domain:[33]

> 48) O Yanis pistevi oti o idios tha kerdhisi
> The John believes that the same FUT win
> "John believes that he (John) will win."
>
> 49) *O Yanis pistevi oti ton eafton tou tha kerdhisi
> "John believes that himself will win."

Note that a literal, idiomatic translation of (48) is impossible because English lacks a comparable feature.

In other words, languages keep the domains of dependent items as separate as possible, and they do so by exploiting the categories (argument domain, minimal domain, maximal domain) created by argument structure. But precisely how each language exploits those categories depends on interactions with other factors, especially the number of dependent referential items the language happens to have.

However, perhaps the most critical problem in binding theory lies in determining not so much the domains within which binding is (im)possible as the circumstances under which constituents in any domain can be bound. A relationship between binding and c-command (varyingly

defined, but the differences between definitions will not concern us here)
has been assumed almost without question for more than two decades.
However, in 1986 a squib by Barss and Lasnik[34] showed that, in double-
object sentences such as (49a):

49a) Mary showed Bill himself in the mirror.

none of the structures hitherto proposed gave the right configuration for
"Bill" to c-command "himself"; indeed, in the most popular and natural of
these structures, "himself" c-commanded "Bill." A number of solutions for
this rather serious problem have been proposed, among them Larsonian
shells[5] and Pesetsky's "cascades,"[35] all of which have been designed to
provide the "right" configuration for c-command to operate.

An attachment framework is free to take a quite different approach.
In fact, what has been called "c-command" falls out from finality of
attachment. Consider the following:

50a) Bill was pleased with himself.

b) Bill's sister was pleased with herself.

c) *Bill's sister was pleased with himself.

The pattern of grammaticality in these sentences is normally attributed
to the fact that the anaphor is c-commanded by "Bill" (50a) or "Bill's sister"
(50b), whereas in (50c), the first branching node that dominates "Bill's"
does not dominate "himself." However, it is equally true that "Bill" and
"Bill's sister" are final attachments in (50a) and (50b), and accordingly bind
anaphors in the minimal domains to which they attach. In (50c), on the
other hand, "Bill's" is not a final attachment – "Bill's" must be attached to
"sister" before "Bill's sister" can be attached to "was pleased . . ." – so "Bill's"
cannot bind the anaphor.

Condition C in classical binding theory ("Referential expressions are
free"), generally attributed to c-command, can also be shown to depend
on order of attachment. Consider (51):

51a) John thinks he lost the key.

b) He thinks John lost the key.

In (51a), "John" and "he" can co-refer; in (51b), they cannot. The reason
is that addition of a final attachment to a minimal domain closes that
domain, rendering it ineligible for many operations. For instance, while
an item lacking independent reference that lies within a closed minimal

domain may (subject to other factors) still be able to get reference from an antecedent in its maximal domain, the reverse is not possible: reference cannot flow outwards and upwards from an antecedent within the closed minimal domain, to a pronoun or anaphor in a maximal domain.

However, none of the above explains the Barss-Lasnik data. For this we must turn to the second basic principle of attachment, priority. In (49), "Bill" is attached first to "showed," and then "himself" is attached to "showed Bill"; "Bill" is therefore a prior attachment with respect to "himself" and within the same minimal domain, therefore binding it by virtue of that priority and domain membership. In (52), however;

<blockquote>52) *Mary showed himself Bill in the mirror.</blockquote>

"himself" is attached prior to "Bill" and therefore cannot bind it, even though, in this case, "Bill" c-commands "himself" (on the most straightforward structural assumptions).

Now consider the following examples:

<blockquote>
53a) I showed the professors each other's students.
b) *I showed each other's students their professors.
54a) I gave every worker his paycheck.
b) *I gave its owner every paycheck.
55a) I gave no-one anything.
b) * I gave anyone nothing.
</blockquote>

Examples (53)-(55) show that anaphoric binding, quantifier scope, and negative scope (all of which supposedly involve c-command) follow an identical pattern in double-object cases; in all of these cases, a prior attachment binds a subsequent one.

In examples (53)-(55), GOALS (datives or indirect objects) precede THEMES (direct objects). It might be suggested that some thematic hierarchy, such as that referred to earlier by Jackendoff, was operative (GOALS can bind THEMES, but not vice versa); den Dikken, although he does not adopt a thematic solution, still finds himself obliged to treat GOAL-THEME and THEME-GOAL constructions differently,[36] because THEME-GOAL examples show an identical pattern to that of (53)-(55):

56a) I introduced the professors to each other's students.

    b) *I introduced each other's students to the professors.

57a) I gave every paycheck to its owner.

    b) *I gave his paycheck to every worker.

58a) I gave nothing to anyone.

    b) *I gave anything to no-one.

However, the present framework can provide a unified treatment for (53)-(58). In every case, regardless whether it is GOAL or THEME, direct or indirect object, the first argument attached binds the second, according to the principle of priority binding.

Two possible alternatives can be quickly disposed of. Although in the cases discussed so far, an initial attachment binds a subsequent attachment, the operative principle is priority rather than initiality, as (59) shows:

59a) Bill sent reminders to John and Mary about each other's birthdays.

    b) *Bill sent reminders to each other about John and Mary's birthdays.

    c) Bill sent reminders about John and Mary's birthdays to each other.

    d) ?*Bill sent reminders about each other's birthdays to John and Mary.

In (59), the initial attachment is of course "reminders," ruling out initiality as the binding factor. Although (59d) is marginally better than (59b), the overall pattern is the same: prior attachments bind subsequent ones, rather than vice versa.

Another alternative that has proved popular over the years[37] has been that of linear precedence: the argument that precedes in linear structure binds the argument that follows. However, this proposal has been rightly rejected by most syntacticians, because syntactic relations are hierarchical rather than linear.

Moreover, the predictions of linear precedence, as well as those of c-command, are violated by cases of so-called "backwards" anaphora, where antecedents that neither precede nor command anaphors still bind them.[38]

60a) Pictures of himself upset Bill.

    b) *Pictures of Bill upset himself.

    c) *Pictures of himself upset Bill's sister.

Again, either priority or finality of attachment accounts for these cases. "Bill" in (60a) is attached prior to "himself." In (60b), "Bill" is part, but not the whole, of the final attachment, and therefore cannot bind; a similar reason disallows (60c), where "Bill" is part, but not the whole, of a prior attachment.

Cases like those of (60) are sometimes regarded as limited to EXPERIENCER predicates. However, as Pesetsky points out,[39] any verb whose subject has a causative (but non-agentive) subject gives similar results:

> 61a) Each other's remarks gave John and Mary a book.
> b) Those books about himself taught Bill the meaning of caution.

Moreover, passive sentences behave similarly:

> 62) The latest rumors about himself have been strongly denied by Clinton.

Of course, with passives it is always possible to posit something like "reconstruction at LF" to account for examples like (62). A similar course is possible in some, but not all cleft sentences, for example (63a), but not (63b).

> 63a) It was himself that Bill criticized.
> b) It was himself that Bill had asked Mary to vote for.
> c) *Bill had asked Mary to vote for himself.

While even on conservative analyses "Bill" can c-command "himself" in (63a) at some stage of the derivation, it is impossible for "Bill" to c-command "himself" without a nearer antecedent, "Mary," also c-commanding it, as in (63c). Thus while c-command will not work without some otherwise-unmotivated reconstruction, priority of attachment within the same domain accounts for all of examples (61)-(63).

Reconstruction, too, fails to give an adequate account of bound variable pronouns. Take the following, for instance:

> 64a) John loved the woman who left him.
> b) The woman who left him loved John.
> 65a) Everyone loved the woman who left him.
> b) *The woman who left him loved everyone.

In order to accommodate examples such as (65b), Chomsky[40] proposed a "Leftness Principle" based on linear order:

66) *A variable cannot be the antecedent of a pronoun to its left.*

However, as Huang[41] points out, even this formulation will not accommodate examples like (67):

> 67a) The woman who loved John decided to leave him ("John" = "him").
> b) *The woman who loved every man decided to leave him ("John" = "him").

Neither (65) nor (67a) presents a problem for the present framework. Bound variable pronouns, like quantifiers, negatives, and anaphors, obey the principles of priority and finality. In (65b), "everyone" is a prior attachment and "him" a constituent of a final attachment, but the situation is not analogous either to that of (60a), where an anaphor in a final attachment is properly bound by a prior attachment, or (51a), where reference flows from a maximal into a minimal domain that is an argument of the maximal domain. (65b) differs from (60a) in that in (65a), the minimal domain of the pronoun is closed by a final attachment ("the woman") and differs from (51a) in that it is not a case of reference flowing from a maximal domain into a minimal domain. The sentence consists of two minimal domains, "The woman who left him" and "[The woman who left him] loved everyone," with constituents inside the square brackets inaccessible to further operations. This is because the verb "left" does not require its final attachment to be sentential (for that matter, no verb does!) so that, no minimal-maximal relationship exists, and the combination of closedness and disjointness of the domains prevents "him" from being bound by "everyone."

Example (67b) is slightly different. Here the antecedent is in the final attachment and the pronoun is an initial attachment (therefore prior to all other attachments). But this configuration merely adds a third factor to the closedness and disjointness of domains that prevented binding in (65b). While final attachments can bind, "every man" forms only part of the final attachment to the minimal domain; this handicap alone would suffice to prevent binding (cf. example [50c] above). Thus although examples like (65) and (67) cannot be handled within other frameworks without extensions of core binding theory, the present framework involves no additional mechanisms.

Note that where priority and finality both obtain, neither overrides the other:

68) John explained Bill to himself.

"Himself" in (68) can be either "John" or "Bill." Still more strikingly, consider (69):

69) John told Bill that pictures of himself were being sold by Sam.

In (69) any of the three arguments "John." "Bill" and "Sam" can bind the anaphor. "Sam" binds by virtue of priority of attachment. "Bill" also binds by priority of attachment, since it is attached to "told" before "that pictures of himself . . ." is attached to "told Bill." "John" binds by virtue of finality; although it is not the final attachment to the minimal domain of "himself." However, because "himself" is itself part of the final attachment to its own minimal domain (thereby excluding the possibility of final attachment binding in that domain), it can be bound by the next final attachment "John."

Let us now consider what might seem to be counterexamples to prior and final binding:

70a) Analysis of herself irritated Susan.
b) *John's analysis of herself irritated Susan.
c) John's analysis of himself irritated Susan.

Why does (70b) fail prior binding? Because complex noun clauses whose heads derive from verbs (plus some that do not, like "picture" phrases, which mimic them) behave exactly like finite or nonfinite clauses: they are argument domains. (70c) is clearly related to "John analyzed himself." If this is the case, then "John's" is clearly the final attachment of a minimal domain, one moreover that is not required by the verb to be sentential. Attachment of a final argument to such a domain closes that domain, preventing coreference between other domain members and outside antecedents. In (70a), on the other hand, the minimal domain "analysis of herself" is not closed by a final attachment; that is, the final argument represented here by the Possessor "John's," has no equivalent, leaving the domain open to prior binding.

It should be noted in this context that complex derived NPs mirror verb-centered argument domains in every respect, showing results in quantifier scope and negative scope as well as in the binding of anaphors:[42]

> 71a) The handing of the toys to each other's creators . . .
>
> b) He handed the toys to each other's creators.
>
> 72a) The clearing of no crumbs off any tables . . .
>
> b) He cleared no crumbs off any tables.
>
> c) *He cleared any crumbs off no tables.
>
> 73a) The plying of each witness with his favorite drink . . .
>
> b) He plied each witness with his favorite drink.
>
> c) *He served his favorite drink to each witness (* unless "He" = "his").

Priority binding handles all these examples without appeal to any (otherwise unmotivated) mechanism. Note further that, because only the attachment of completed arguments, rather than those arguments' internal structure, counts in the present framework, the fact that many of these are PPs rather than NPs or DPs (which creates problems for any analysis relying on c-command) is quite irrelevant here.

A rather different type of structure is exhibited in (74):

> 74a) I consider a fear of each other John and Mary's greatest problem.
>
> b) *I consider a fear of John and Mary each other's greatest problem.

At first sight, this seems like a clear violation of priority. A subsequent attachment appears to bind a prior one, while the predicted configuration fails to bind. However, the two arguments "a fear of X and Y" and "X and Y's greatest problem," are not in fact arguments of "consider," but arguments of a small clause, which in turn is a reduction of finite and nonfinite clauses of similar meaning:

> 75a) I consider John a fool.
>
> b) I consider John to be a fool.
>
> c) I consider that John is a fool.

In (74a), therefore, "John and Mary's greatest problem" attaches first to a copula with zero phonetic representation,[43] and accordingly has priority over the final attachment "a fear of each other." In (74b), in contrast, the anaphor attaches first, and even though "John and Mary" occurs in the final attachment, it is not the whole of that attachment, therefore cannot bind through finality. Because no other potential binder is available, the sentence is ungrammatical.

A different type of problem is presented by sentences like (76):[44]

> 76) Sue showed each other's friends to John and Mary.

Here, a prior attachment seems to be bound by a subsequent one. But there are two things to be taken into consideration here. First, the structure of (76) is identical to that of (56b), which many writers,[45] including myself, regard as ungrammatical. Second, in (76) (as for that matter in [56b]), the anaphor is not a prior attachment, but a part of such an attachment (it is attached to "friends" in [76], and to "students" in [56b], before being attached to the main structure of the sentence). Thus such cases are clearly marginal as compared with cases in which the anaphor, as well as a prior attachment, is itself an argument (e.g., [52], which is uncontroversially ungrammatical). Clearly something is going on here that has to do with differences between prior and final attachments, and between attachment within an argument as specifier as opposed to attachment as complement. This needs to be clarified by further research (see discussion of doubtful cases at the end of this section).

A case where varying informant judgements would seem not to be involved concerns the contrast between (77a) and (77b):

> 77a) ?Each other's criticisms harmed John and Mary.
> b) *Each other's parents harmed John and Mary.

While (77a) is dubious, the contrast between (77a, b) seems clear enough. "Each other" binding suggests a cline of acceptability from sentences like (61a) through sentences like (77a) to sentences like (77b). It would seem here that a semantic differential, involving a progressively stronger degree of agency, is involved, as well perhaps as the specifier/complement distinction referred to in the previous paragraph. It may be that final attachments to final attachments have a status different from that of complements to final attachments; again, only further investigation will clarify the issue.

Many dubious cases involve sentences in which both antecedent and anaphor are non-arguments. Where both are arguments, results are always clear. When one is an argument and the other a nonargument, results are almost always clear, save for the kind of semantic issues shown in (77). When both are nonarguments, however, judgements can much more readily be influenced by semantic or even pragmatic factors, which can override the normal inability of a nonargument to bind an anaphor:

> 78a) Relatives of the bride and groom thought each other's stories were hilarious.
>
> b) Attorneys for the twins thought each other's alibis were phoney.

The two sentences are identical in structure, but in (78a), the natural reading is that the relatives thought each other's stories were hilarious, rather than that relatives of the groom thought the bride's stories hilarious and relatives of the bride thought the groom's stories hilarious. However, in the very different context of (78b), it is perhaps more plausible to suppose that the attorney for twin A thought twin B's alibi was phoney while the attorney for twin B thought twin A's alibi was phoney, rather than that the two attorneys thought each other's alibis were phoney.

A similar example is (79):

> 79) Bill and Mary's stories made each other's friends suspicious.

Because stories do not have friends, "each other" can more readily be taken to corefer with "Bill and Mary." However, part of the problem lies in the very different statuses of "self" anaphors and "each other." The distribution of these as nonarguments is quite different; "himself" can only be a prior attachment (Comp) while "each other" can be either a final attachment (Spec) or a prior attachment. This may be connected with the fact that while there are pronominal equivalents for all "self" anaphors, there is no pronominal (that is, no nonreferential item free in its own domain) that corresponds with "each other." In consequence, "each other" sentences (provided there is a possible plural antecedent somewhere in the sentence) are likelier, other things being equal, to be judged grammatical than "self" sentences.

However, insofar as apparent counterexamples to the present proposal are either supportive of it (when correctly analyzed) or involve marginal cases influenced by semantic considerations, we can conclude that the principles of priority and finality give a coverage of scope and binding problems that is surprisingly broad, especially considering the restrictiveness of the mechanisms invoked.

Accordingly, we may state conditions on binding as follows:

80a) *Anaphors are bound by prior attachments and/or by the nearest final attachment.*

b) *Pronouns are free in their minimal domains.*

Conclusion

IN THE FOREGOING SECTIONS, several of the main aspects of syntax have been discussed, including argument structure, government, the mapping of argument structure to phrase structure, movement, barriers to movement, empty categories, binding and co-reference, scope, and c-command. It has proved possible to account for major features in all these areas through the minimal primitives (A) through (D). The fact that this is possible, and that a grammar arising from research into the evolution of language combines such extensive coverage with such extremely restrictive principles, strongly suggests that language evolution did indeed follow the paths that we have proposed in the body of this book.

———————————————

Glossary

The **bold face terms** are cross-references to other glossary items; the ALL-CAPS ITEMS are the roles in argument structure. Many technical linguistic terms will not be found here, e.g., for "empty categories," consult the index and the appendix.

There is a more extensive neuro glossary in *The Cerebral Code*, available at *http://WilliamCalvin.com/bk9gloss.html*. The present glossary is also on the web at *http://WilliamCalvin.com/LEMglossary.html*.

AGENT   A role *(the performer of an action)* in **argument structure** (*JOHN* cooked dinner).

allele   Alternative versions of a **gene**. Perhaps 20 percent of your expressed genes have a different allele on the other chromosome; that is, you are *heterozygous* for that gene and might switch to using it under some conditions. One reason that hybrids don't breed true to type is that parents are often passing on their less-used allele. Inbred strains have less heterozygosity.

altruism   Doing something for another's benefit, at expense to yourself – but not necessarily at the expense of your genes, as when you aid relatives. In reciprocal altruism (RA), sharing with nonrelatives is eventually reciprocated, though the system is weakened by freeloaders ("cheaters").

area   When capitalized, it's a *Brodmann Area*, a subdivision of cerebral cortex based on the relative thickness of the six layers. Area 17 is better known as primary visual cortex; it seems to be a functional unit, but Area 19 comprises at least six major functional units. A territory or work space is a generic lower-case area, occupied temporarily by active patterns of cloned hexagons.

argument structure The assignment of **thematic roles** to the constituents (noun-phrases, prepositional phrases, even clauses) that represent the participants in actions, states, and events creates *arguments*. Some of these arguments are obligatory, depending on the meaning of the verb. Argument structure is what determines whether a verb will have one, two or three obligatory arguments. Thus, "sleep" will have only one, a sleeper. "Break" will have two, a breaker and something broken. "Give" will have three, a giver, a gift, and a receiver. Unlike **phrase structure**, argument structure does not assign either linear ordering or hierarchical relationships to its components; argument structure has to be mapped onto phrase structure in order to provide these.

axon   The neuron's tail-like "wire," a long (0.1 - 2,000 mm), spider thread thin portion of the neuron that carries voltages between the neuron's input sites (concentrated on cell body and dendritic tree) and the neuron's outputs, its many-branched axon terminals that make synapses onto downstream neurons. It's typically a one-way street, messages flowing from the dendrites and cell body to the far end of the axon where synapses are made.

bee dance The honeybee appears, at least in the context of a simple coordinate system, to have broken out of the usual animal communication that has a single meaning. When the bee returns to her hive, she performs a "waggle dance" in a figure-8 that communicates information about the location of a food source that she has just visited. The angle of the double racetrack's common axis communicates the direction of the new-found food, and the number of circuits that she does around the loops communicates the distance from the hive. But, as Bickerton said in *Language and Species*,

> All other creatures can communicate only about things that have evolutionary significance for them, but human beings can communicate about *anything*.... Animal calls and signs are structurally holistic [and] cannot be broken down into component parts, as language can.... Though in themselves the sounds of [human] language are meaningless, they can be recombined in different ways to yield thousands of words, each distinct in meaning.... In just the same way, a finite stock of words... can be combined to produce an infinite number of sentences. Nothing remotely like this is found in animal communication.

BENEFICIARY   A role *(doing something for someone)* in **argument structure** (I bought it *FOR YOU*).

binding   Binding theory describes the conditions that identify constituents without independent reference – pronouns and anaphors (reflexives, reciprocals, and the like). See the appendix.

bonobo   *Pan paniscus*, formerly called the "pygmy chimpanzee," and the last great ape species to be identified. Until 1927, they were confused with the chimpanzee, *Pan troglodytes* – with the old common name arising because they were said to be the "chimpanzee of the pygmies," living as they do on the left bank of the Congo River in equatorial forests (they're called the "Left Bank Chimps" for other reasons, too). While of a more slender body build than chimps, bonobos are not particularly smaller. Humans last shared a common ancestor with both *Pan* species about 5 million years ago. The two *Pan* species diverged at about the beginning of the ice ages, 2.5 million years ago, roughly the same time that the *Australopithecus* lineage spun off the *Homo* lineage.

bottleneck   In population biology, an occasion when genetic variability in a population was greatly simplified by the loss of alternative **alleles** – not because of selection against them but simply due to dropouts that occur by chance, because of reduced choice in mates. This happens when population numbers are greatly reduced for a time; the re-expansion then populates the world from the smaller range of variation.

central nervous system (CNS) The brain, spinal cord, and the retina (all the rest is the peripheral nervous system).

cerebral cortex The outer 2 mm (that's two thin coins worth) of the brain's cerebral hemispheres with a layered structure. It isn't required for performing a lot of simple actions but seems essential for creating new episodic memories, the fancier associations, and many new movement programs. Paleocortex, and archicortex such as hippocampus, has a simpler structure and earlier evolutionary appearance than the six-plus-layered **neocortex**.

cheater detection A feature of reciprocal **altruism** theories, what you use to identify freeloaders who receive but rarely give back.

chunking Collapsing multiple-word phrases into a single word, in the manner of acronyms.

clause   A verb and all its associated arguments. See **phrase**.

code   In cryptography, a *code* is a disguising transformation that (unlike a *cipher*) also chunks – and thereby shortens – the message, as when a number stands for a standard five-word phrase. More generally, as in genetic code, *code* refers to the transformation of a representation's short form into its long-form implementation. As such, it is analogous to a matrix. *Code* may also simply refer to the short form itself, such as a DNA base-pair sequence capable of generating a particular protein.

columns   A minicolumn is a cylindrical group of about 100 neurons about 0.023 mm in diameter, extending through all the layers of **neocortex** and usually organized around a dendritic bundle; the orientation column is an example. Macrocolumns are a hundred times larger in area (and about 0.4 -1.0 mm across) and often more like curtain folds than cylinders; they are typically identified by common inputs, e.g., the ocular dominance columns of visual cortex.

corticocortical connection   An **axon** or axon bundle connecting one patch of cerebral cortex to another. Some remain local, within the superficial layers of cortex, while others go tunneling through the white matter to distant targets – some, via the corpus callosum, to the other cerebral hemisphere.

creole   Children invent a new language – a creole – out of the words of the pidgin **protolanguage** they hear their immigrant parents speaking. A **pidgin** is what traders, tourists, and "guest workers" (and, in the old days, slaves) use to communicate when they don't share a real language; pidgin sentences are unstructured and short, while those in creoles have the features of **universal grammar**.

Darwin Machine   The Calvin 1987 coinage, on the Turing Machine analogy, for any full-fledged Darwinian process incorporating the six essentials for the Darwinian algorithm. Species evolution, the immune response, some genetic algorithms, and the hexagonal work space competitions are all examples. Not to be confused with particular models, also named after Darwin.

dendrite   Neurons have branches. At least in neocortex, dendrites are the receiving branches of the neuron and the axon is the sending branch. Elsewhere, some dendrites can also act like axon terminals, releasing **neurotransmitter** in response to impulses and local voltage changes. There is always a single thin **axon** that initiates and propagates **impulses** to distant destinations, and there are somewhat thicker dendritic branches that receive **synapses** from other neurons's axon terminals. Pyramidal neurons have a tall tree-like *apical dendrite* plus some rootlike *basal dendrites.*

epigenetic rules Some aspects of development are both innate and specified by the environment; "epigenetic" applies to the environmental bits. For example, a plant has two growth states, a positively phototaxic mode that directs most growth toward the light, and a negatively phototaxic mode. Some vines initially grow away from the light; then, when there is enough root structure, further growth is up towards the light; the vine climbs any tree trunk and its branches. Then some vine tips turn negatively phototaxic, dropping a branch down to earth which, upon reaching soil, digs in to create another set of roots. The behavioral switch may be provided by **genes**, but the overall form of the resulting plant also depends upon what was encountered in the environment along the way. **Syntax** too is likely to have epigenetic aspects; the sign-language-deprived deaf infants might be like plants with only oblique light.

exaptation This was a term intended to cover cases where an organ with one original function got adapted to perform another function (such as the swim-bladders becoming lungs when the first marine creatures became terrestrial). Previously, the term "pre-adaptation" had been used, but this form is objectionable insofar if it suggests some degree of prescience. (WHC: I use it anyway.)

gene A unit of heredity, essentially that segment of a DNA molecule comprising the code for a particular peptide or protein. We also talk loosely of "a gene for blue eyes" and so forth (reification strikes again), but many a DNA gene is pleiotropic: it has multiple (and sometimes very different) effects on its body; like that maxim about intervening in complex systems, "You can't do just *one* thing."

genotype The full set of genes carried by an individual, whether expressed or silent **alleles**. Similar to *genome*. Compare to *phenotype*. What makes living matter so different from other self-organizing systems is that a cell has an information center, the genes, concerned with orchestrating the many different processes going on within the cell, and in such a manner that copies of the cell tend to survive.

GOAL   A role *(whoever the action was directed toward)* in **argument structure** (I gave it *TO MARY*).

grammar   Not to be confused with socially correct usage. In order to handle novel sentences, we not only need to access the words stored in our brains but also the patterns of sentences possible in a particular language. These patterns describe not just patterns of words but also patterns of patterns. There are three aspects of grammar: morphology (word forms and endings), **syntax** (from the Greek "to arrange together" – the ordering of words into clauses and sentences), and phonology (speech sounds and their arrangements). A complete collection of rules is called the mental grammar of the language, or grammar for short.

grammar, universal   Each of the languages of the world has a corresponding mental grammar, constructed as we learn the language. Though they differ in many ways, the human brain seems to have a highly specific menu of possibilities for grammatical organization, known as Universal Grammar, or UG, that structures language learning even when the input itself is lacking in structure (pidgins, home sign, and so on).

grammatical morphemes   The words (a few dozen in English) that refer to relations between content words. They are unlike content words, which refer to concepts of things in the world. They include words that express relative location (*above, below, in, on, at, by, next to*), relative direction (*to, from, through, left, right, up, down*), relative time (*before, after, while*, and the various indicators of tense), and relative number (*many, few, some*, the *-s* of plurality). The articles express a presumed familiarity or unfamiliarity (*the* for things the speaker thinks the hearer will recognize, *a* or *an* for things the speaker thinks the hearer won't recognize) in a manner somewhat like pronouns. Others express relative possibility (*can, may, might*), relative contingency (*unless, although, until, because*), possession (*of*, the possessive version of *-s, have*), agency (*by*), purpose (*for*), necessity (*must, have to*), obligation (*should, ought to*), existence (*be*), nonexistence (*no, none, not, un-*), and so forth. These are called "closed-class words" because our ways of expressing relationships are so resistant to augmentation, whereas you can always create new nouns or verbs.

head See **phrase**.

impulse *Action potential* and *spike* are synonyms; an impulse is the regenerative change in the voltage across the neuron's membrane used for long-distance (more than a millimeter) signaling in the nervous system. It is brief (1/1000 sec, quicker than any other signal in the brain but a million times slower than computers) and large (only 1/10 volt but bigger than any other voltage in the brain). Its threshold property can also be used as a simple decision making mechanism. See also **axon, myelin**.

inflections The inflectional system of English alters a noun when it refers to a multiplicity (*"The boy ate three cookie."* Is that correct English?) and alters a verb when it refers to past time (*"Yesterday the girl pet a dog."* OK?). Late learners of English may fail to realize that anything is "wrong" with these incorrect sentences, as such long-range dependencies are redundant information that helps out in noisy environments when some words are imperfectly heard and must be guessed.

innateness "Hardwired by genes" is the general idea, but it is, more generally, a bit of behavior that arises without learning. When the individual finds itself in a particular setting, out pops some complicated behavior. Mating behaviors are innate; some things are too important to be left to learning. But there isn't a dichotomy between innateness and environmental causation; as **epigenetic rules** show, something innate may have, via environmental triggers, profound effects on future form and function.

INSTRUMENT A role (*doing it with something*) in **argument structure** (Bill cut it *WITH A KNIFE*).

irregular An irregular noun does not follow the usual plural rule. By the age of two or three, children learn to add *-s*. Before that, they treat all nouns as irregular. But even if they had been saying "mice," once they learn the plural rule they may begin saying "mouses" instead. Eventually they learn to treat the irregular nouns as special cases, exceptions to the usual rule. Verbs too can be irregular: the past tense of "fly" is "flew" – unless, of course, the word is being used in some novel manner, as in "The batter *flied out*," where the regular *-ed* form is nonetheless used. Young children, however, often use the regular form for the central meaning of "fly," as in "The bird flied away."

inheritance principle Darwin's great but often misunderstood insight, that variation is not truly random. Rather than variations being done from some ideal or average type, small undirected variations are preferentially done from the more successful individuals of the current generation, exploring the solution space nearby (not jumping randomly to somewhere truly unrelated) in the next generation. [?]

island biogeography The peculiarities of animal and plant species when largely isolated, with just occasional interbreeding. An "island" can also be a deep ocean basin, a high mountain valley, or a patch in a patchy resource distribution that prevents migration. Islands often have a reduced number of species, so traditional predators or parasites may be lacking. Species often arrive in small numbers, so bottlenecks are a standard feature of island populations.

language acquisition device The LAD is a hypothetical mechanism in the human brain that enables any normal human to learn any of the 5000+ human languages (or any possible human language). Its existence has never been empirically demonstrated and, within the present approach, it would seem to be unnecessary to assume any LAD as a distinct, self-encapsulated unit.

meme Richard Dawkins's 1976 coinage, on the analogy to **gene** (with a little aid from mime and mimic), for a cultural copying unit, such as the word or melody that is mimicked by others.

memory, dual trace Hebb's 1949 coinage for separate systems implementing short- and long-term memories: active (spatiotemporal) and passive (spatial-only) memory traces.

memory, episodic One-trial learning involving distinct episodes, such as being an eyewitness to an accident. Such memories are notoriously malleable, influenced by subsequent events and the mistakes made in earlier recall attempts.

movement Where a word moves out of its usual place in a sentence, as in the *wh-* words. See the appendix.

myelin   The fatty, porcelain-colored insulation around an **axon** that reduces its energy consumption while also making the impulse travel much faster. It is wrapped in layers, like a bandage.

neocortex All of **cerebral cortex** except for such things as hippocampus, the simpler layered structure that lacks the patterned recurrent excitatory connections and columnar structures that make the six-layered neocortex so interesting.

nervous system The whole works, both **central nervous system** (CNS: brain, spinal cord, and retinas) and peripheral nervous system (most sensory and muscle connections, plus the clusters of neurons called ganglia).

neuron   The nerve cell, whether sensory neuron, interneuron, or motor neuron. There are about 10^{12} neurons in the human brain and spinal cord; the neocortex alone is said to have 10^{11}. The *cell body* of the neuron is the widest section, thanks to containing the cell nucleus, and there are many processes branching off, receiving inputs and distributing outputs. See **dendrite, axon**.

neurotransmitter A molecule such as glutamate or acetylcholine that is released from an axon terminal (often by the arrival of an **impulse**), diffuses across a narrow extracellular space, and binds with a receptor on the surface of the **postsynaptic** cell. (These three parts are collectively called the **synapse**).   Many dozens of neurotransmitters have been identified over the years, and a given axon terminal may release more than one kind.

niche   The "outward projection of the needs of an organism" such as food resources, migration routes, camouflage from predators, suitable housing and sites for effective reproduction. An *empty niche* is a proven niche space that is temporarily unoccupied by a tenant species.

parcellation   Fragmentation; breaking apart a population into smaller, isolated units ("parcels" or "patches"), as when rising sea level converts a hilly island into an archipelago of former hilltops. See also **island biogeography**.

PATIENT   A role *(who- or whatever undergoes the action)* in **argument structure** (John cooked *DINNER*). Often described as THEME.

phenotype   Usually "body" but actually the entire constitution of an individual (anatomical, physiological, behavioral) resulting from the interaction of the genes with the environment. As Dawkins emphasized in *The Extended Phenotype*, can even include such things such as bird nests.

phoneme   The units of vocalization distinguished by native speakers of a language. Unlike ape calls and cries, phonemes are all meaningless by themselves, having meaning only in combinations (words). It is important to realize that phonemes are categories that standardize. For example, Japanese has a phoneme that is in between the English /L/ and /R/ in sound space.   Those English phonemes are mistakenly treated by Japanese speakers as mere variants on the Japanese phoneme.   Because of this "capture" by the familiar category, those Japanese speakers who can't hear the difference will also pronounce them the same, as in the familiar rice-lice confusion.

phrase   A group of words consisting of a *head* (which can be a noun, verb, preposition, etc.) and its *modifiers.* **Clauses** consist of groups of phrases. Each phrase is labeled according to its head. If the head is a noun, the phrase will be a *noun phrase* ("the tall blond man," where "man" is the head). If the head is a preposition, the phrase will be a *prepositional phrase* ("with one black shoe," where the head is "with").

phrase structure   The results of the procedure by which words and phrases are assembled to form clauses and sentences. Formerly an independent module in generative grammar, its features now fall out from the principles that govern other modules. However, *phrase structure trees* are still drawn by syntacticians to show the relationships between words, phrases, and clauses. Such trees are hierarchically structured and, nowadays, usually binary-branching.

pidgin   A contact medium liable to spring up wherever speakers of several different languages have to communicate without any language in common. In its early stages of development a pidgin is a form of **protolanguage**: that is to say, it lacks any kind of formal structure. Pidgin utterances consist of small groups of content words strung together in a purely ad hoc fashion. A pidgin, if it endures long enough, may stabilize, expand and, after several generations, approach the status of a full natural language. If a pidgin, regardless of its stage of development, is acquired by children, they convert it into a **creole**.

postsynaptic   The postsynaptic neuron's dendrite receives neurotransmitter, rather in the manner of sniffing perfume, and changes the permeability of its membrane to certain ions, usually Na^+, K^+, Cl^-, or Ca^{++} in some combination. Ions flowing through the membrane in turn produce the voltage change known as the *postsynaptic potential* (PSP). If excitatory, it is called the EPSP; if inhibitory, the IPSP.

protolanguage   Any form of communication that contains arbitrary, meaningful symbols but lacks any kind of syntactic structure. Forms of protolanguage include the communication of "linguistically"-trained apes and other animals, **pidgins** in their early stages, the speech of nonproficient second-language learners, and that of children under two.

pyramidal neurons   The excitatory **neurons** of neocortex. They typically have a tall apical **dendrite** (an exception is the spiny stellate neuron) and a triangular-shaped cell body (from whence the name), from which their **axon** leaves. The neurons contributing to the pyramidal tract (alias the corticospinal tract, named for the triangular shape of the axon bundle as it traverses the medulla) are themselves pyramidal neurons, but most pyramidal neurons send axons elsewhere.

receptive field   A map of the inputs to a single **neuron**, e.g., those parts of the skin of the hand that produce excitation or inhibition of a cortical neuron (antagonistic surrounds are especially common). The limited view of the world as seen by a single neuron. [?]

recombination   There are several connotations: (1) The shuffling of genetic material between an individual's two chromosome pairs that occurs just prior to the production of ova or sperm (the crossing-over phase of meiosis); and (2) the production of a new individual through the union of a sperm and an ovum from two parents at fertilization.

schema   As in "schematic outline," it's a mental item more abstract than a rich mental image of an object. In some cognitive contexts, it is used more narrowly for those things like *more, less, bigger, inside* – things grounded in our everyday experiences, often making reference to our own body moving through our daily world. Movements need something similar, and schema is often used to refer to standard movement programs.

semantics   The "meaning" of words, those connotations that you might look up in a dictionary (as opposed to **syntax**).

SOURCE   A role *(taking it from someone or something)* in **argument structure** (I bought it *FROM FRED*).

synapse   The synapse is the junction between neurons across which communications flow, usually in the form of *neurotransmitter* molecules secreted by the *presynaptic* axon terminal that diffuse a short distance across the extracellular space (the *synaptic cleft*) to the *postsynaptic* neuron, on whose membrane are some receptor molecules to which the neurotransmitter molecules reversibly bind. While they are bound, they open up an ion channel through the postsynaptic membrane, producing postsynaptic current flow. Most drugs affecting the **CNS** operate by interfering with synaptic transmission. See also **dendrite, neuromodulator, neurotransmitter, postsynaptic.**

syntax   The set of rules and principles that determine how sentences are formed, and the structures resulting from sentence formation.

THEME   A role *(who- or whatever undergoes the action)* in **argument structure** (John cooked *DINNER*).

UG   See **grammar, universal**.

word order   A simple convention that aids in identifying roles, such as the subject-verb-object order (SVO) of most declarative sentences in English ("The dog bit the boy") or the SOV of Japanese. At least in English, the who-what-where-when-why-how questions deviate from basic word order: "What did John give to Betty?" is the usual convention (except on quiz shows in which questions mimic the basic word order and use emphasis instead: "John gave *what* to Betty?"). Some languages such as Latin lack a systematic word order, instead using characteristic inflections or even separate words (as when

English uses "he" for a subject and "him" for an object, although both have singular, masculine, third-person referents) to help disambiguate the sentence.

Notes

Short-form citations such as DENNETT (1996) either refer to the authors' books below or to a nearby full-length citation. The bibliography for the appendix is at the end.

DEREK BICKERTON, *Roots of Language* (Karoma, 1981).

DEREK BICKERTON, *Language and Species* (University of Chicago Press, 1990).

DEREK BICKERTON, *Language and Human Behavior* (University of Washington Press, 1995).

WILLIAM H. CALVIN, *How Brains Think: Evolving Intelligence, Then and Now* (Basic Books, 1996a).

WILLIAM H. CALVIN, *The Cerebral Code: Thinking a Thought in the Mosaics of the Mind* (MIT Press, 1996b).

WILLIAM H. CALVIN and GEORGE A. OJEMANN, *Conversations with Neil's Brain: The Neural Nature of Thought and Language* (Addison-Wesley, 1994).

These books also likely contain citations to many of the items we do not document below.

Chapter 1. The Villa Serbelloni

page

vi ERNST MAYR, *This is Biology* (Harvard University Press, 1997), p. 158.

4 "The idea that our prize possession, language, is just some mechanical thing . . . ." See, for example, MICHAEL BEAKEN, *The Making of Language* (University of Edinburgh Press, 1996), where the author rejects generative grammar because it does not concern itself with the social use of language, or PHILIP LIEBERMAN, *Eve Spoke: Human Language and Human Evolution* (W.W. Norton, 1998), which describes Chomskyan linguistics as "toy linguistics" (p. 125).

4 For an interesting review of Chomsky's remarks on language and evolution, see FREDERICK J. NEWMEYER, "On the supposed counterfunctionality of Universal Grammar: some evolutionary implications" in JAMES R. HURFORD, MICHAEL STUDDERT-KENNEDY and CHRIS KNIGHT, *Approaches to the Evolution of Language* (Cambridge University Press, 1998).

5 "Some of what has been written . . . ." DEREK BICKERTON, "I chat, thereby I groom." *Nature* 380:303 (1996).

7 "Stages in child's development...." C. DARWIN, "A biographical sketch of an infant," *Mind*, July, 1877, pp. 285-294, reprinted in *Developmental Medicine and Child Neurology*, v. 13, n. 5, supplement 24, 1971, pp. 1-8.

10 "Nine new words every day...." STEVEN PINKER, *The Language Instinct* (Allen Lane, London, 1994), p. 151.

11 SVEN BIRKERTS, *The Gutenberg Elegies: The Fate of Reading in an Information Age* (Faber and Faber 1994). "Not only is the text a distillation, a dramatic shaping of materials, but the... result is an altered state of awareness, a kindled-up sort of high."

Chapter 2. What Are Words?

13 For discussion of the relationship between words and what they signify, see ROGER BROWN, *Words and Things* (Harvard University Press, 1970), and WILLARD QUINE, *Word and Object* (Wiley and Sons, 1960).

15 FERDINAND DE SAUSSURE, *Course in General Linguistics* (McGraw-Hill, 1966 [1915]).

15 "the picture of reality you carry about . . . ." I have dealt with these issues at some length: BICKERTON (1990), see especially Chapters 2 and 4.

16 The idea that words have properties that have to match if the words are to be combined, is central to Chomsky's Minimalist Program. NOAM CHOMSKY, "A minimalist program for linguistic theory" in KENNETH HALE and SAMUEL JAY KEYSER, eds., *The View from Building 20: Essays in Linguistics in Honor of Sylvain Bromberger* (MIT Press, 1993), pp. 1-52.

See also NOAM CHOMSKY, "Bare phrase structure", in GERT WEBELHUTH, ed., *Government and Binding Theory and the Minimalist Program: Principles and Parameters in Syntactic Theory* (Basil Blackwell, 1995), pp. 383-439.

19 "what makes cartoon sketches so successful...." SCOTT MCCLOUD, *Understanding Comics: The Invisible Art* (Kitchen Sink Press, 1993).

19 Themes, see GERALD HOLTON, "On the art of scientific imagination," *Daedalus* 125(2):183-208 (Spring 1996).

For looking at things with a Darwinian template, see my examples in W. H. CALVIN, "The Six Essentials? Minimal Requirements for the Darwinian Bootstrapping of Quality.," *Journal of Memetics - Evolutionary Models of Information Transmission*, 1 (1997), at *http://www.fmb.mmu.ac.uk/jom-emit/1997/-vol1/calvin_wh.html*.

20 DOROTHY L. CHENEY and ROBERT M. SEYFARTH, *How Monkeys See the Worlds: Inside the Mind of Another Species* (University of Chicago Press, 1990).

20 "when a chimpanzee drags a branch." See ELLEN J. INGMANSON, "Tool-using behavior in wild *Pan paniscus*: Social and ecological considerations," in ANNE E.

RUSSON, KIM A. BARD, and SUE TAYLOR PARKER, eds., *Reaching into Thought: The Minds of the Great Apes* (Cambridge University Press, 1996), pp. 190-210 at p. 201.

21 Direct continuity of animal calls and language has a long history and a wide representation in the literature. For a proposal more concrete (if no more plausible) than most, see CHARLES F. HOCKETT and ROBERT ASCHER, "The human revolution," *Cultural Anthropology* 5:135-168 (1964). A more recent, more tentative, and more sophisticated approach is that of MARC D. HAUSER, *The Evolution of Communication* (MIT Press, 1996).

23 TERRENCE DEACON, *The Symbolic Species: The Co-evolution of Language and the Brain* (W.W. Norton, 1997).

23 For details about the chimpanzee Sherman, see E. SUE SAVAGE-RUMBAUGH, *Ape Language: From Conditioned Response to Symbol* (Columbia University Press, 1986).

For a recent account of Kanzi, see SUE SAVAGE-RUMBAUGH, STUART G. SHANKER, and TALBOT J. TAYLOR, *Apes, Language, and the Human Mind.* (Oxford University Press, 1998).

24 "the real rubicon," HERBERT S. TERRACE, LOUISE A. PETITTO, ROBERT J. SANDERS and THOMAS G. BEVER, "Can an ape create a sentence?" *Science* 206:891-900 (1979).

25 T. J. GRABOWSKI, HANNA DAMASIO, and ANTONIO R. DAMASIO, "Premotor and prefrontal correlates of category-related lexical retrieval," *Neuroimage* 7:232-243 (1998).

HANNA DAMASIO, T. J. GRABOWSKI, DANIEL TRANEL, R. D. HICHWA, and ANTONIO R. DAMASIO, "A neural basis for lexical retrieval," *Nature* 380:499-505 (1996).

Chapter 3. Why Putting Words Together Isn't Easy

28 ROBERT M. W. DIXON, ed., *Grammatical Categories in Australian Languages* (Australian Institute of Aboriginal Studies, 1976).

29 For the one-word stage in language acquisition, see LOIS BLOOM, *One Word at a Time: The Use of Single Word Utterances before Syntax* (Mouton, 1973).

29 Typical samples of protolanguage can be found in the appendix to BICKERTON 1995.

30 "depart from the customary word-order unpredictably . . . ." In other words protolanguage varieties do not, unlike true languages, move words for specific reasons, such as to give them added emphasis.

30 A more positive view of protolanguage is given in discussion of the "pragmatic mode" by TALMY GIVON, *On Understanding Grammar* (Academic Press, 1979).

30 Of course you'll point out here that toddler talk *does* develop into true language. Or does it? Might it not be the case that true language simply *replaces* toddler talk? (More about this in the appendix.)

32 For instance, Genie – see SUSAN CURTISS, *Genie: A Psycholinguistic Study of a Modern-Day "Wild Child"* (Academic Press 1977) – who was raised without language by her abusive father until she was thirteen, and never passed beyond the protolanguage stage despite falling well within the normal IQ range and undergoing intensive instruction for several years (for a full discussion see BICKERTON 1990).

32 PATRICIA K. KUHL, S. KIRTANI, T. DEGUCHI, A. HAYASHI, E. B. STEVENS, C. D. DUGGER, and P. IVERSON, "Effects of language experience on speech perception: American and Japanese infants' perception of /ra/ and /la/," *Journal of the Acoustical Society of America* 102:3135 (1997).

32 PINKER (1994), p. 151.

33 For a comprehensive description of how pidgin-to-creole conversion happened in Hawaii, see SARAH J. ROBERTS. "The role of diffusion in the genesis of Hawaiian Creole." *Language* 74 (1998).

JUDY KEGL and GAYLE A. IWATA, "Lenguage de Signos Nicaraguense: a pidgin sheds light on the 'creole'?", in ROBERT CARLSON et al., eds., *Proceedings of the Fourth Meeting of the Pacific Linguistics Conference,* 266-294 (Department of Linguistics, University of Oregon, 1989) describes a similar situation among the deaf in Nicaragua.

33 Some of the erroneous structures we impose on chaos happen to be useful, e.g., even though we first viewed electrons as circling the atom's nucleus like a planet, it was a useful stepping-stone to quantum mechanics' probabilistic cloud.

37 URSULA BELLUGI, P. P. WANG, and T. L. JERNIGAN, "Williams' syndrome: an unusual psychoneurological profile." In S. BROSNAN and J. GRAFMAN, eds., *Atypical Cognitive Deficits in Developmental Disorders: Implications for Brain Function,* 23-56 (Erlbaum, 1994).

38 DOREEN KIMURA, *Neuromotor Mechanisms in Human Communication* (Oxford University Press 1993).

GEORGE A. OJEMANN, "Cortical organization of language," *Journal of Neuroscience* 11:2281-2287 (August 1991); "Cortical organization of language and verbal memory based on intraoperative investigations," *Progress in Sensory Physiology* 12:193-230 (1991).

Chapter 4. Bigger than a Word, Smaller than a Sentence

41 For a fuller discussion of the differences between protolanguage and language, see BICKERTON 1990.

41 Unfortunately, I know of no really good, really simple introduction to syntax – the world badly needs one. Chapter 4 of STEVEN PINKER, *The Language Instinct* (William Morrow & Co., 1994) is more fun than most.

43 Speed differences, cited in BICKERTON 1983.

45 Just about any work on generative grammar later than about 1980 will discuss empty categories. None of these books are what you'd call easy reading; the most user-friendly one that I know is ANDREW RADFORD, *Transformational Grammar: A First Course* (Cambridge University Press, 1988).

47 Of course, in answers to questions, we may find isolated phrases (say, "his new credit card") if the question was something like "What did Fred put into his wallet?" But this merely presupposes that the structure of the question is somehow present in the answer, and many linguists believe that "Fred put . . . in his wallet" was present at an earlier phase of composing the sentence and subsequently removed prior to utterance.

48 PINKER (1994), p. 86.

48 The pioneer in argument structure was JEFFREY S. GRUBER, whose 1965 doctoral dissertation, *Studies in Lexical Relations*, was published in 1970 by the Indiana University Linguistics Club. Since then there have been literally hundreds of publications dealing with thematic roles and argument structure, among which RAY JACKENDOFF, *Semantic Interpretation in Generative Grammar* (MIT Press, 1972) is one of the more readable and widely quoted works.

50 Of course, you will find sentences like "Bill kicked and struggled, but could not escape his assailants." Many transitive verbs have intransitive equivalents, but there's a big difference here between "kicked" and "struggled": you can have "Bill kicked his assailants" but not "Bill struggled his assailants." You have to say, "Bill struggled WITH his assailants." And the reason you have to include the preposition is that "struggle" is a REAL intransitive, not – like "kick" – a transitive that on occasion will allow actions that don't reach or maybe don't even have targets.

50 MICHEL DEGRAFF (personal communication) points out that there are verbs like "bet" or "wager" that (it could be argued) involve four obligatory participants:"I (*1*) bet you (*2*) five dollars (*3*) that the Falcons win the Super Bowl (*4*)." However, since "I bet you that the Falcons win the Super Bowl" is a perfectly grammatical sentence, the insertion of a sum of money appears (although heavily favored in our culture) to be optional. Similarly, one can say "Bill bet fifty bucks that Rabid Chomskyite would win in the fifth." It would be bizarre, even if factually accurate, to say "Bill bet the bookie fifty bucks."

50 Imperatives might seem an obvious exception to this. If I say "Get out!", no participant at all is expressed. Yet neither is any ambiguity involved. "Get out!" means that whoever I am addressing should get out – not the cat, or the President, or anyone else, but "You!"

51 "For every invisible argument there's a visible argument in the same sentence that refers to the same person or thing." This is oversimplifying a little. Generic arguments may be there without overt form or any antecedent. For instance, if I say "They sang for an hour," it can be understood that what they sang were songs, not short stories or telephone directories. Similarly, if I say "To get there is real easy," I mean it's easy for anyone to get there.

Chapter 5. Language in the Brain

The basic reference for chapters 5-8 is *The Cerebral Code*, though the last two chapters of *How Brains Think* cover the topics more briefly, as does W. H. CALVIN, "Competing for consciousness: A Darwinian mechanism at an appropriate level of explanation," *Journal of Consciousness Studies* 5(4):389-404 (1998). They are available at *http://WilliamCalvin.com* on the web.

57 Neurologists have a somewhat maddening tendency to write about language as if it were words ("Language gives us names for things") and maybe sentences, often missing the point that syntax is our best example of how structured thinking works. Nonetheless, let me strongly recommend Antonio R. Damasio's *The Feeling of What Happens* (Harcourt Brace, 1999) which tackles the whole spectrum of consciousness quite usefully, including how language amplifies it (*http://WilliamCalvin.com/1990s/1999NYTBR.htm*).

58 GREGORY BATESON: "Information is a difference that makes a difference." He noted that data is just a signal of a difference. (With thanks to Stewart Brand.)

58 "[often] information from the sense organs and our memories is being collected in aid of a plan of action." In deciding whether to order expensive or risky medical tests, physicians have to ask themselves whether the results are likely to help them decide what to do next. And that depends on the treatment options (often, getting a brain scan makes no practical difference) or if there are dangerous alternative diagnoses to rule out.

59 For more on concept categories revealed by strokes, see the last chapter of CALVIN & OJEMANN (1994).

59 JOHN HART and BARRY GORDON, "Neural subsystems for object knowledge," *Nature* 359:60-64 (1992). Offers evidence for a major division between visually-based and language-based higher-level representations.

60 Human temporal lobe concepts, see ANTONIO R. DAMASIO and DANIEL TRANEL, "Nouns and verbs are retrieved with differently distributed neural systems," *Proceedings of the National Academy of Sciences (U.S.A.)* 90:4957-4760 (1 June 1993).

Chapter 6. How Are Memories Stored?

67 HENRY DAVID THOREAU (Bradley P. Dean, editor), *Faith in a Seed : The Dispersion of Seeds and Other Late Natural History Writings* (Island Press, 1993), at p. 12.

69 Not only was the Canadian psychologist D.O. HEBB amazingly ahead of his time with the concepts in *The Organization of Behavior* (Wiley 1949), but so was the English biologist J. W. S. PRINGLE with his paper, "On the parallel between learning and evolution," *Behaviour* 3:174-215 (1951). I thank Richard Dawkins for bringing Pringle's work to my attention and Greg Ransome for noting FRIEDRICH HAYEK'S *The Sensory Order* from the same period.

Chapter 7. Hexagonal Mosaics and Darwin Machines

For more background on copying competitions, see W. H. CALVIN, "The Six Essentials? Minimal Requirements for the Darwinian Bootstrapping of Quality," *Journal of Memetics - Evolutionary Models of Information Transmission*, 1 (1997), at *http://www.fmb.mmu.ac.uk/jom-emit/1997/vol1/calvin_wh.html*.

75 SANTIAGO RAMÓN Y CAJAL, *Recuerdos de mi Vida: Historia de mi Labor Científica* (Madrid: Alianza Editorial, 1923).
81 "Many models of coupled oscillators exhibit such entrainment." ARTHUR WINFREE, "Biological rhythms and the behavior of populations of coupled oscillators," *Journal of Theoretical Biology* 16:15-42 (1967).

Chapter 8. A Common Code: The Brain's "Esperanto" Problem

100 EDWARD O. WILSON, *Consilience* (Harvard University Press, 1998).
102 R. SHADMEHR and H. H. HOLCOMB, "Neural correlates of motor memory consolidation," *Science* 277:821 (8 August 1997).

Chapter 9. Protolanguage Emerging

103 There are any number of good books about evolution, so we're not going to rehash the basics of this subject. Anyone who wants a good, accessible summary could read RICHARD DAWKINS, *The Blind Watchmaker* (Longmans, 1986) or STEPHEN JAY GOULD, *Wonderful Life* (W.W. Norton, 1989). For a more academic approach, see GEORGE C. WILLIAMS, *Adaptation and Natural Selection* (Princeton University Press, 1966).
103 For an account of the progressive increase of human brain size, see PHILIP V. TOBIAS, *The Brain in Hominid Evolution* (Columbia University Press, 1971) and TERRENCE W. DEACON, *The Symbolic Species* (Norton, 1997).
103 ROBERT FOLEY (1987). "Hominid species and stone tool assemblies," *Antiquity* 61:380-392. Contains a comparison between the stone tools of various ancestral species.
105 A summary of the Caldwell's studies of signature whistles can be found in M. C. CALDWELL, D. K. CALDWELL AND P. TYACK, "Review of the signature whistle hypothesis for the bottlenosed dolphin", in S. LEATHERWOOD and R. R. REEVES, eds., *The Bottlenosed Dolphin* (Academic Press, 1990).

105 FRANS DE WAAL, *Chimpanzee Politics: Power and Sex among Apes* (Johns Hopkins University Press, 1998).

106 JANE GOODALL, *The Chimpanzees of Gombe* (Harvard University Press, 1986); GEORGE B. SCHALLER, *The Mountain Gorilla: Ecology and Behavior* (University of Chicago Press, 1963); BARBARA B. SMUTS, *Sex and Friendship in Baboons* (Aldine, 1986).

106 "alliances, altruism, cheating, loyalty, revenge, betrayal." FRANS DE WAAL, *Good-natured: The Origin of Right and Wrong in Modern Humans* (Harvard University Press, 1996).

107 NICHOLAS K. HUMPHREY, "The social function of intellect," in P. G. BATESON and R. A. HINDE, eds., *Growing Points in Ethology* (Cambridge University Press, 1976), 303-317.

107 RICHARD W. BYRNE and ANDREW WHITEN, *Machiavellian Intelligence: Social Expertise and the Evolution of Intellect in Monkeys, Apes and Humans* (Oxford University Press, 1988).

107 DAVID PREMACK and GEORGE WOODRUFF, "Does the chimpanzee have a theory of mind?" *Behavioral and Brain Sciences* 4:515-526 (1978).

107 CECILIA M. HEYES, "Theory of mind in nonhuman primates," *Behavioral and Brain Sciences* 21:101-148 (1998) provides a recent and thorough overview of this somewhat contentious field.

108 "a prerequisite for language as we know it." See, for example, ROBERT WORDEN, "The evolution of language from social intelligence," in HURFORD, STUDDERT-KENNEDY and KNIGHT, eds. (1998), pp. 148-166.

108 The literature on teaching symbolic systems to apes is now enormous. It falls roughly into three phases, one of extreme optimism (BEATRIX T. GARDNER and R. ALAN GARDNER, "Teaching sign language to a chimpanzee," *Science* 165:664-672 (1969), then one of pessimism (HERBERT S. TERRACE, *Nim* [Knopf 1979]), then one of more careful and cautious rebuilding (SAVAGE-RUMBAUGH 1986).

110 So far as we know, band size, even as late as the Paleolithic, was quite small. See F. A. HASSAN, *Demographic Archaeology* (Academic Press, 1981), who suggests that the average group size at that time was as little as 22 (with a range from 11 to 31).

111 See ROBERT FOLEY, *Another Unique Species* (Longman Group, 1987), for a good account of early hominid ecology.

111 CHENEY and SEYFARTH (1990, pp. 283-286). The authors carried out ingenious experiments with the carcasses of leopard kills and artificial python tracks, to which vervet monkeys failed entirely to respond. They also report naturalistic observations in which monkeys ignored clear signs that predators were close by, reacting only when the predator itself appeared.

111 According to PAUL R. EHRLICH, *The Machinery of Nature* (Simon and Schuster, 1986), in the Serengeti, hyenas obtain about 33 percent of their food from scavenging, lions and leopards 10 percent-15 percent, and hunting dogs 3 percent; among hunting predators, only cheetahs refrain from scavenging.

115 STEPHEN JAY GOULD and RICHARD C. LEWONTIN, "The spandrels of San Marco and the Panglossian paradigm: a critique of the adaptationist program,"*Proceedings of the Royal Society B* 205:581-598 (1979).

115 "Wraaa!", see JANE GOODALL, *The Chimpanzees of Gombe* (Harvard University Press, 1986), p. 127.

116 It has even been suggested, quite seriously, that language evolved so that men out hunting all day could ask relatives or neighbors if their wives had been unfaithful to them in their absence (MATT RIDLEY, *The Red Queen*, Macmillan, 1993, p. 229, citing an interview with Richard Wrangham).

116 SUE SAVAGE-RUMBAUGH, STUART G. SHANKER AND TALBOT J. TAYLOR, *Apes, Language, and the Human Mind* (Oxford University Press, 1998), p. 60.

117 "[N]ames for basic-level object kinds are among the first words acquired and are considerably more frequent in child language than they are for adults," according to PAUL BLOOM, "Theories of word learning: rationalist alternatives to associationist," in WILLIAM C. RITCHIE and TEJ K. BHATIA, *Handbook of Child Language Acquisition* (Academic Press, 1999), 249-278 (citation from p. 254). Even though other words learned early include things that do not indicate simple objects, these, according to Bloom, consist mainly of features of the environment such as "beach," "kitchen," "sky," "rain," "morning," and so on.

118 ELINOR OCHS, *Culture and Language Development: Language Acquisition and Language Socialization in a Samoan Village* (Cambridge University Press, 1988); BAMBI SCHIEFFELIN, *The Give and Take of Everyday Life: Language Socialization of Kaluli Children* (Cambridge University Press, 1990).

119 Kanzi pointing, see p. 56 of SUE SAVAGE-RUMBAUGH, "Why are we afraid of apes with language?" pp. 43-69 in *The Origin and Evolution of Intelligence*, edited by ARNOLD B. SCHEIBEL and J. WILLIAM SCHOPF (Sudbury MA: Jones and Bartlett, 1997).

120 "major facts about hunting." The list is mine but, for a serious backgrounder, see MATT CARTMILL, *A View to a Death in the Morning* (Harvard University Press, 1993).

For some of the changing views of paleoecology, see RICHARD W. WRANGHAM, JAMES HOLLAND JONES, GREG LADEN, DAVID PILBEAM, NANCYLOU CONKLIN-BRITTAIN, "The raw and the stolen: cooking and the ecology of human origins," *Current Anthropology* (to appear, 1999).

120 "rather than simply snatching the prize." See RICHARD WRANGHAM, DALE PETERSON, *Demonic Males: Apes and the Origins of Human Violence* (Houghton Mifflin, 1996).

121 ERNST MAYR, *This is Biology* (Harvard University Press, 1997), pp. 184-185.

Chapter 10.
Reciprocal Altruism as the Predecessor of Argument Structure

123 "I and others." Syntax, see TERRENCE et al. (1979).

124 Sexual selection, see HELENA CRONIN, *The Ant and the Peacock* (Cambridge University Press, 1992).

124 ANITA DAUGHERTY, *Marine Mammals of California* (State of California Dept. of Fish and Game, 1972).

125 "neocortex size." RICHARD W. BYRNE, *The Thinking Ape: Evolutionary Origins of Intelligence* (Oxford University Press, 1995).

B. PAWLOWSLI, ROBIN I. M. DUNBAR, and C. LOWEN, "Neocortex size, social skill and mating success in male primates," *Behaviour* 135: 357-368 (1998).

125 "genes of others preferential treatment." WILLIAM D. HAMILTON, "The genetical evolution of social behavior," *Journal of Theoretical Biology* 7:1-52 (1964).

125 ROBERT TRIVERS, "The evolution of reciprocal altruism," *Quarterly Review of Biology* 46:35-57 (1971).

126 "as many subsequent ethological studies confirmed." For example, SHIRLEY C. STRUM, *Almost Human: A Journey into the World of Baboons* (Random House, 1987); DE WAAL (1996, 1998).

127 Social life references, see Chapter 4 notes.

127 Friendships, from STRUM (1987), p. 135 (emphasis added).

128 Subtle cheater, from STEVEN PINKER, *How the Mind Works* (W.W. Norton, 1997) p. 403.

130 DAVID I. PERRETT, M. H. HARRIES, R. BEVAN, S. THOMAS, P. J. BENSON, A. J. MISTLIN, A. J. CHITTY, J. K. HIERANEN and J. E. ORTEGA, "Framework of analysis for the neural representation of behavior", *Journal of Experimental Biology* 146:87-113 (1989).

130 See ENDEL TULVING, "Elements of episodic memory," *Behavioral and Brain Sciences*, 7:223-238 (1984) and commentaries thereon for a variety of views on the nature of memory.

DAVID S. OLTON, "Comparative analysis of episodic memory," *Behavioral and Brain Sciences* 7:250-251 (1984).

WHC: Remember that the links between different elements of an episodic memory may become unreliable. See ELIZABETH F. LOFTUS, "Creating false memories," *Scientific American* 277(3):70-75 (September 1997) and her *Eyewitness Testimony* (Harvard University Press, 1996).

133 Group selection backsliding, see ELLIOTT SOBER and DAVID SLOAN WILSON, *Unto Others: The Evolution and Psychology of Unselfish Behavior* (Harvard University Press, 1998).

134 And why might altruism flourish in a climatically-challenged sub-population? See chapter 13 and W. H. CALVIN, "The emergence of intelligence," *Scientific American Presents* 9(4):44-51 (November 1998). Available at *http://WilliamCalvin.com/1990s/1998SciAmer.htm.*

Chapter 11. Role Links for Words

136 Exaptation was a term coined by STEPHEN JAY GOULD and ELISABETH S. VRBA, "Exaptation – a missing term in the science of form," *Paleobiology* 1:4-15 (1982).

137 "language began as . . . ." BICKERTON (1990, 1995).

138 The parentheses around NP and E merely mean that these elements are optional – a verb-phrase could consist of just the verb, as in "Bill left."

139 "Argument can be rewritten as . . . ." For simplicity I ignore optional arguments here. Their presence or absence makes no difference with respect to what's at issue.

140 Most natural word order, see BICKERTON (1981).

140 The process described here, discussed at greater length in the appendix, is similar to the process called "Merge" which is central to Chomsky's most recent work: NOAM CHOMSKY, "Bare phrase structure", in GERT WEBELHUTH, ed., *Government and Binding Theory and the Minimalist Program* (Basil Blackwell, 1995), pp. 383-439.

141 See JOSEPH GREENBERG, *Language Universals: With Special Reference to Feature Hierarchies* (Mouton, 1976) to get some idea of the variety of different ways in which languages can map argument structure onto syntax.

144 For Darwinian aspects, see CALVIN (1996); GERALD EDELMAN, *Neural Darwinism* (Basic Books, 1987); DANIEL DENNETT, *Consciousness Explained* (Little, Brown & Co., 1991).

145 Some linguists – for example, DAVID PESETSKY, *Zero Syntax* (MIT Press, 1995) – would surely disagree, and (in Pesetsky's case) claim that we also need EXPERIENCER (for the subjects of "psychological" verbs like "consider" or "fear," and CAUSER for things that have causative effects but can't be regarded as conscious, deliberate AGENTS. Such linguists may well be right, but even if they are, it makes no difference to my present argument.

146 ROBERT J. RICHARDS, *Darwin and the Emergence of Evolutionary Theories of Mind and Behavior* (University of Chicago Press, 1987), p. 399.

148 "what I formerly conceived as a single step." DEREK BICKERTON, "Catastrophic evolution: the case for a single step from protolanguage to full human language," in JAMES R. HURFORD, MICHAEL STUDDERT-KENNEDY and CHRIS KNIGHT, eds., *Approaches to the Evolution of Language* (Cambridge University Press, 1998), 341-358.

148 For more details on Tokpisin, see GILLIAN SANKOFF, "The genesis of a language," in KENNETH C. HILL, ed., *The Genesis of Language* (Karoma, 1979).

150 WHC: Let me mention some next-level-up categories that Derek's categorical roles suggest to me, often called image schemas in cogsci (see TURNER 1996, p. 16). They're not just for objects but also for actions. *Motion along a path* is a simple image schema, used for locomotion, reaching out, falling apples, pouring tea, and so forth. Simple ones can combine to form a complex one, as when the *goal* of a *path* is said to be the *interior* of a *container*. It doesn't take a motor systems neurophysiologist like me to recognize that "force dynamics" provides a lot of schemas for us to use at higher-than-concrete levels, e.g., *pushing, pulling, resisting, yielding, releasing, dipping, rising, climbing, falling*, and the aforementioned *pouring*.

Things like this aren't as fundamental as AGENT, THEME, GOAL – you won't complain about a sentence being ungrammatical if they're missing or overdetermined – but they might well be part of the higher levels above the social calculus roles, when we make small stories and then larger stories out of the morass of our experience.

167 I borrowed the Jewish Buddhist mantra from my friend Peter Warshall.

Chapter 12.
The Word Tree as a Secondary Use of Throwing's
Segmented Movement Planner

The basic background on accurate throwing's challenges is W. H. CALVIN, "The unitary hypothesis: A common neural circuitry for novel manipulations, language, plan-ahead, and throwing?" In *Tools, Language, and Cognition in Human Evolution*, edited by Kathleen R. Gibson and Tim Ingold (Cambridge University Press,1993), pp. 230-250.

153 For the misleading illusion of the little person inside, see DANIEL C. DENNETT, *Consciousness Explained* (Little, Brown, 1991) and ANTONIO R. DAMASIO, *The Feeling of What Happens* (Harcourt Brace, 1999).

154 WILLIAM JAMES, "Great men, great thoughts, and the environment," *The Atlantic Monthly* 46(276):441-459 (October 1880).

163 Now that children develop the brain's structured planning machinery before the age of three, well before *accurate* throwing is practiced, it may be that adult throwing operates somewhat differently now than it did earlier in evolution, simply because throwing is now the secondary use of the structured neural machinery rather than vice versa. Practicing prepositions could now affect the way accurate throwing is practiced!

168 MARK TURNER, *The Literary Mind* (Oxford University Press, 1996), p. 47.

168 FYODOR MIKHAILOVICH DOSTOEVSKY, *Notes From Underground [Letters from the Underworld]* (1864). Searchable at *http://kuyper.cs.pitt.edu/d/dostoevsky/underground/-underground11.txt*.

Chapter 13.
Corticocortical Coherence Promotes a
Many-Voiced Symphonic Sentence

The long version of corticocortical coherence is in Chapter 8 of *The Cerebral Code*, available at *http://WilliamCalvin.com/bk9/bk9ch8.htm* on the web.

169 JACOB BRONOWSKI, *The Origins of Knowledge and Imagination* (Yale University Press 1978, transcribed from 1967 lectures), p. 105.

175 Dropping back to an incoherent arcuate fasciculus is something of a model for disconnection syndromes such as Wernicke's conduction aphasia. What's usually described as conduction aphasia is a stroke that doesn't obviously damage auditory cortex or Wernicke's area, one which largely affects white matter such as arcuate fasciculus. That doesn't mean that it gets all (or even most) of the arcuate fasciculus. Strokes that are bigger are also likely to damage the aforementioned cortical areas, and therefore get called something else. So conduction aphasia is almost by definition a small stroke.

The main deficits described for what gets labeled conduction aphasia are repetition difficulties (and even that is denied by some authors) and paraphasias for words. Broca's and Wernicke's areas are what light up in PET on working memory tasks such as rehearsing a phone number long enough to dial it, so this likely involves arcuate. What would really hurt structured sentences of some complexity, in my model, would be functional disorganization of the arcuate, e.g., sprouting secondary to injury, timing changes because of disrupted myelination, etc. – not fractional loss of arcuate per se.

179 TURNER (1996), p. 20.
182 TURNER (1996), p. 57.

Chapter 14. The Pump and the Slingshot

183 DANIEL C. DENNETT, *Kinds of Minds: Toward an Understanding of Consciousness* (Basic Books, 1996), p. 147.
185 Concealed ovulation, see JARED DIAMOND, *Why is Sex Fun?* (Basic Books, 1997).

274

186 W.H. CALVIN, "The great climate flip-flop," *The Atlantic Monthly* 281(1):47-64 (January 1998). See also *http://faculty.washington.edu/wcalvin/1990s/-1998AtlanticClimate.htm*.

187 An extensive bibliography on abrupt climate change can be found at *http://WilliamCalvin.com/climate/* on the web.

190 W.H. CALVIN, "A stone's throw and its launch window: timing precision and its implications for language and hominid brains," *Journal of Theoretical Biology* 104:121-135 (1983).

W. H. CALVIN, "The unitary hypothesis: A common neural circuitry for novel manipulations, language, plan-ahead, and throwing?" in *Tools, Language, and Cognition in Human Evolution*, edited by KATHLEEN R. GIBSON and TIM INGOLD (Cambridge University Press, 1993), pp. 230-250.

190 One example of a relaxation is in the size of the human chewing teeth. As food preparation involving pottery is discovered, there is a drop of 10 to 15 percent in the surface area of the cheek teeth. This happens at different times in different parts of the world, but all correlate with when food technology improvements occur. See C. LORING BRACE, KAREN R. ROSENBERG, and KEVIN D. HUNT, "Gradual change in human tooth size in the late Pleistocene and post Pleistocene." *Evolution* 41:705-720 (1987). Another relaxation is probably nearsightedness. (At least, I have difficulty imagining a hunting-and-gathering population with the modern percentage of myopia!)

192 OLIVER SACKS, *Seeing Voices* (University of California Press, 1989).

193 FRANS DE WAAL, *Good Natured: The Origins of Right and Wrong* (Harvard University Press, 1996).

193 ALBERT EINSTEIN (inscription on his statue in front of the National Academy of Sciences, Washington DC, USA).

Chapter 15. Darwin and Chomsky Together at Last

196 FRIEDRICH MAX MULLER, *Lectures on the Science of Language delivered at the Royal Institute of Great Britain in April, May and June, 1861*, 4th ed. (Longman, Green, Longman, Roberts and Green, 1864), p. 368.

196 "from inarticulate cries." CHARLES DARWIN to Max Muller (3 July 1873), in *More Letters of Charles Darwin*, FRANCIS DARWIN, ed. (Appleton, 1903) 2: 45.

196 Ban: Societe Linguistique de Paris, *Statuts*, Section 2 (1886).

197 EMIL KRAEPELIN's major works, ignored for decades, have been translated and reprinted, e.g., *Lectures in Clinical Psychiatry*, THOMAS JOHNSTONE, ed. (Hafner, 1968 – facsimile of 1904 edition); *Manic Depressive Insanity and Paranoia* (Arno Press, 1976 – reprint of 1921 edition).

197 NOAM CHOMSKY, *Cartesian Linguistics: A Chapter in the History of Rational Thought* (Harper and Row, 1966). Reasons for this Cartesian choice are far from clarified by Chomsky's most recent discussion of it ("Knowledge of history and theory construction in modern linguistics," *Revista de Documentacao de Estudoes em Linguistica Teorica e Aplicada*, vol 13, Numero Especial, 1997, pp. 103-122).

200 Of course, nowadays apes suffer under a far more remorseless pressure than human ancestors ever had to contend with: us. But we weren't around when the nature of modern apes was being forged, and though it would be nice to see them mutate fast and develop defensive strategies (even weapons), there's not the slightest chance that they will.

202 HERBERT G. WELLS, "The Grisly Folk," in *Selected Short Stories of H.G. Wells* (Penguin Books, 1958), pp. 285-298; WILLIAM GOLDING, *The Inheritors* (Harcourt, Brace & World, 1955).

205 Although we still don't know much more than generalities about *why* the brain enlarged, we increasingly know something about what changed in development to produce a larger brain/body ratio. See TERRENCE W. DEACON, *The Symbolic Species* (Norton, 1997) for the story.

205 DEREK BICKERTON, "Creole languages, the language bioprogram, and language acquisition" in WILLIAM C. RITCHIE and TEJ K. BHATIA, eds., *Handbook of Child Language Acquisition* (Academic Press, 1999), pp. 195-220.

205 For a description of the syntactic spurt, see WILHELM LEOPOLD, *Speech Development of Bilingual Child* (Northwestern University Press, 1939-1949), Vol. 4; and JOHN LIMBER, "The Genesis of Complex Sentences," in JOHN MOORE, ed., *Cognitive Development and the Acquisition of Meaning* (Academic Press, 1973), pp. 169-185.

206 Recapitulationist idea: ERNST HAECKEL, *Anthropogenie oder Entwicklungsgeschichte des Menschen* (Engelman, 1891).

See, for example, DAVID POEPPEL and KENNETH WEXLER, "The full competene hypothesis of clause structure in early German," *Language* 69:1-33 (1993).

An extensive survey of the consequences of Broca's aphasia in several languages can be found in LISA MENN and LORRAINE K. OBLER, *Agrammatic Aphasia: A Cross-Language Narrative Textbook* (Benjamins, 1990, 3 vols.).

210 MYRNA GOPNIK and M. B CRAGO, "Familial aggregation of a developmental language disorder," *Cognition* 39:1-50 (1991).

Linguistics Appendix: Notes

page, [note number] (*name-year* references are in the bibliography that follows these notes)

216 [1] Chomsky (1995), p. 386.

216 [2] Chomsky's citation[1] could be interpreted in this light; for an even clearer statement, see Lightfoot (1997).

216 [3] Theory underdetermined by data: more generally, see Chomsky (1966).

216 [4] Chomsky (1995); see also Marantz (1995).

217 [5] Larson (1988). See the criticism of his proposals by Jackendoff (1990).

217 [6] Pollock (1989). See the criticism of his proposals by Iatridou (1990).

217 [7] For instance, those cited in Barss and Lasnik (1986).

217 [8] It dates from Reinhart (1976), and is thus among the oldest surviving generative mechanisms.

218 [9] There is no mention of "Merge" in Chomsky (1993) or even Marantz (1995); the notion emerges only in Chomsky (1995, but published as an Occasional Paper the previous year).

218 [10] Chomsky (1997, p. 191).

219 [11] Chomsky (1997, p. 191).

219 [12] Chomsky (1986). See also Reinhart and Reuland (1993).

220 [13] See Vergnaud (1974), Kayne (1994). As will be shown below, this analysis does not require to be stipulated within the present framework; it follows necessarily from the attachment process.

221 [14] Chomsky (1981).

222 [15] That all branching must be binary was originally proposed by Kayne (1984).

222 [16] Chomsky (1995), p. 397.

223 [17] Abney (1987).

224 [18] Chomsky (1995, pp. 395-398).

225 [19] In this respect, the present proposals follow the Universal Alignment Hypothesis of Perlmutter and Postal (1984) rather than the Uniformity of Theta-Assignment Hypothesis (Baker 1988).

225 [20] This discussion benefits from, even if it does not exactly follow, the discussion in Pesetsky (1995, Chapters 2 and 3).

226 [21] Note a similar alternation with some of the Theme/Experiencer cases noted in the preceding paragraph:

    i)   Politics worries John
    ii) John worries about politics
    iii) Ghosts frighten John
    iv) John is frightened of/by ghosts

This suggests that when a causative-type verb moves its Experiencer to final attachment, the demoted Theme/Cause moves and requires a preposition (see discussion of passive, below).

226 [22] There have been numerous attempts to establish a thematic role hierarchy, for a variety of purposes. See for example Jackendoff (1972) and Randall (1984), among others. Interestingly, although it was designed for binding purposes, Jackendoff's

hierarchy (AGENT > GOAL > THEME) is virtually identical with the one described here. In discussing it, Williams (1995, p. 122) noted that the implied connection between binding theory and theta theory was a "surprising" one. The observation is just, but if we assume that both binding and theta-role mapping are determined by a single factor – priority and finality of attachment – the connection no longer surprises.

226 [23] Compare with the treatment of "chomage" in Perlmutter (1971).

227 [24] There are some obvious exceptions, such as

> i) John was said by Bill to have been arrested EC.

where A-movement carries "John" right outside its minimal domain. However, even if gaps and traces are assumed here, the same mechanism used to identify ECs left by A bar movement (see below) works equally well.

227 [25] cf., Chomsky (1995), Kayne (1994).

228 [26] The description of the copy theory of movement by Marantz (1995, 373) could hardly be improved on, and is accepted here without reservation. What is really interesting about this proposal is that in all probability the brain performs exactly as the theory would predict. While the brain is assembling a sentence (presumably by means of some complex signal coded for all the sentence constituents), the part of the signal that encodes a moved constituent must appear in both (original and target) positions; there would seem no other, certainly no simpler way of establishing coreference. However, the motor control areas must be somehow instructed which of the two copies must be given phonetic form and which must be ignored.

228 [27] Note, however, that adjunct phrases of time, place, etc., can be attached directly to the node dominating the final attachment:

> i) In the afternoon Mary works in her garden.

However, many languages (such as German) require licensing by a tensed auxiliary for any postfinal attachment, which is what leads to the existence of so-called V2 languages.

230 [28] cf. Chomsky (1981, pp. 195, 231-233). The example given is from Hornstein and Weinberg (1995, p. 268, ex. 74a).

232 [29] e.g., Pesetsky (1989); Rizzi (1990).

235 [30] See Lasnik (1976), Chomsky (1980), Higginbotham (1980), Reinhart (1983), Manzini and Wexler (1987), and Pollard and Sag (1992) for a representative sampling of varied approaches to binding.

236 [31] Chomsky (1981).

236 [32] According to Carden and Stewart (1988).

236 [33] Details and examples from Iatridou (1986).

237 [34] Details and examples from Iatridou (1986).

237 [35] Pesetsky (1995).

238 [36] den Dikken (1995, pp. 216-217). The details of his proposals do not concern us here; briefly, they involve a cascade-type structure for Goal-Theme structures and A-movement for Theme-Goal structures.

239 [37] Langacker (1969) was among the first to suggest that linear precedence played a role in binding. The suggestion has been raised more recently by Barss and Lasnik (1986) and Jackendoff (1990), among others.

239 [38] Examples are from Williams (1989).

240 [39] Pesetsky (1995, p. 201).

240 [40] Chomsky (1976).

241 [41] Huang (1995, pp. 140-1).

243 [42] These examples are from Pesetsky (1995, p. 186).

243 [43] To regard small clauses as systematic reductions of copula clauses is, of course, only one of many solutions in the literature for the problem presented by small clauses. Moreover, it is not a viable solution for many small clauses:

 i) *They ate the meat was raw.
 ii) *They elected Bill is president.

although "They elected/chose Bill to be president" is possible. Although it would be nice to give all small clauses a single analysis (and many treatments attempt just this), there is no logical reason why they should all share the same structure. In this context it is worth noting that many languages, in particular many creoles, have separate copulas for NP_NP and NP_Adj environments (the second being usually zero, with the adjective behaving in many ways like a verb, see Bickerton 1973).

244 [44] This example is from Pesetsky (1995, p. 222).

244 [45] For instance, den Dikken (1995, p. 217) and Barss and Lasnik (1986).

Linguistics Appendix: Bibliography

Abney, S. 1987. The English noun phrase in its sentential aspect. Doctoral dissertation, MIT.

Baker, M. 1988. *Incorporation: A theory of Grammatical Function Changing.* Chicago: University of Chicago Press.

Barss, A., and H. Lasnik. 1986. A note on anaphora and double objects. *Linguistic Inquiry* 17.347-354.

Bickerton, D. 1973. The nature of a creole continuum. *Language* 49.640-669

Bralich, P. 1991. Doctoral dissertation, University of Hawaii.

Carden, G., and W.A. Stewart. 1988. Binding theory, bioprogram and creolization: evidence from Haitian Creole. *Journal of Pidgin and Creole Languages* 3.1-69.

Chomsky, N. 1965. *Cartesian Linguistics: A Chapter in the History of Rational Thought.* New York: Harper and Row.

Chomsky, N. 1976. Conditions on rules of grammar. *Linguistic Analysis* 2.303-351.

Chomsky, N. 1980. On binding. *Linguistic Inquiry* 11.1-46.

Chomsky, N. 1981. *Lectures on government and binding.* Dordrecht: Foris.

Chomsky, N. 1986. *Knowledge of language: Its nature, origin and use.* New York: Praeger.

Chomsky, N. 1993. A minimalist program for linguistic theory. In K. Hale and S.J. Keyser, eds., *The View from Building 20: Essays in Linguistics in Honor of Sylvain Bromberger*, pp. 1-52. Cambridge, Mass.: MIT Press.

Chomsky, N. 1993. Bare phrase structure. In G. Webelhuth, ed., 381-439.

Chomsky, N. 1997. Interview in *Chomsky no Brasil: Revista de Documentacao de Estudos em Linguistica Teorica e Aplicada*, Vol. 13, Special Number, 159-193.

den Dikken, M. 1995. *Particles: on the syntax of verb-particle, triadic, and Causative constructions.* Oxford: Oxford University Press.

Higginbotham, J. 1980. Pronouns and bound variables. *Linguistic Inquiry* 11.679-708.

Hornstein, N., and A. Weinberg. 1995. The empty category principle. In G. Webelhuth, ed., 241-296.

Huang, C.-T. J. 1995. Logical form. In G. Webelhuth, ed., 125-175.

Iatridou, S. 1986. An anaphor not bound in its governing category. *Linguistic Inquiry* 17.766-772.

Iatridou, S. 1990. About Agr(P). *Linguistic Inquiry* 21.551-577.

Jackendoff, R. 1972. *Semantic Interpretation in Generative Grammar.* Cambridge, Mass.: MIT Press.

Jackendoff, R. 1990. On Larson's treatment of the double object construction. *Linguistic Inquiry* 21.427-456.

Kayne, R. 1984. *Connectedness and Binary Branching.* Dordrecht: Foris.

Kayne, R. 1994. *The Antisymmetry of Syntax.* Cambridge, Mass.: MIT Press

Langacker, R. 1969. Pronominalization and the chain of command. In D. Reibel and S. Schane, eds., *Modern studies in English.* Englewood Cliffs, N.J.: Prentice-Hall.

Larson, R. 1988. On the double object construction. *Linguistic Inquiry* 19.33-91.

Lasnik, H. 1976. Remarks on coreference. *Linguistic Analysis* 2.1-22.

Lightfoot, D.W. 1997. Reply to Bauer. *Language* 73.358.

Manzini, M.R., and K. Wexler. 1987. Oarameters, binding theory and learnability. *Linguistic Inquiry* 18.413-444.

Marantz, A. 1995. The minimalist program. In G. Webelhuth, ed., 349-382.

Perlmutter, D. 1977. *Deep and Surface Structure Constraints in Syntax.* New York: Holt, Rinehart and Winston.

Perlmutter, D.M, and P. Postal. 1984. The I-advancement exclusiveness law. In D.M. Perlmutter and C. Rosen, eds., *Studies in Relational Grammar 2*, 81-125. Chicago: University of Chicago Press.

Pesetsky, D. (1989). Language-particular processes and the Earliness Principle. Ms, MIT, Cambridge, Mass.

Pesetsky, D. 1995. *Zero syntax: Experiencers and cascades.* Cambridge, Mass.: MIT Press.

Pollard, C., and I. Sag. 1992. Anaphors in English and the scope of binding theory. *Linguistic Inquiry* 23.261-303.

Randall, J.H. 1984. Thematic structure and inheritance. *Quaderni di Semantica* 5.92-110.

Reinhart, T. 1976. The syntactic domain of anaphora. Doctoral dissertation, MIT.

Reinhart, T. 1983. Coreference and bound anaphora: a restatement of the anaphora question. *Linguistics and Philosophy* 6.47-88.

Reinhart, Tanya, and Eric Reuland. 1993. Transitivity. *Linguistic Inquiry* 17.501-558.

Rizzi, L. 1990. *Relativized minimality.* Cambridge, Mass.: MIT Press.

Vergnaud, J.-R. 1974. French relative clauses. Doctoral dissertation, MIT.

Webelhuth, G. (ed.) 1995. *Government and binding theory and the minimalist program: Principles and parameters in syntactic theory.* Oxford: Basil Blackwell.

Williams, E. 1989. The anaphoric nature of theta-roles. *Linguistic Inquiry,* 20.425-456.

Williams, E. 1995. Theta theory. In G. Webelhuth, ed., 97-124.

The Authors

WILLIAM H. CALVIN

I majored in physics at Northwestern University (B.A., 1961), spent a year at M.I.T. and Harvard Medical School absorbing the atmosphere of what eventually became known as neuroscience, then went to the University of Washington to do a degree in physiology and biophysics (Ph.D., 1966) working under Charles F. Stevens. I subsequently stayed in Seattle, on the faculty of the Department of Neurological Surgery, a wonderful postdoctoral education as well as a home for my experimental work on neuron repetitive firing mechanisms, from lobster neurons *in vitro* to human cortical neurons *in situ*. After a 1978–79 sabbatical as Visiting Professor of Neurobiology at the Hebrew University of Jerusalem, my interests began to shift toward theoretical issues in the ensemble properties of neural circuits – what eventually became Darwin

Machines – and to the big brain problem of hominid evolution. Friends in psychology, zoology, archaeology, and physical anthropology tried hard to educate me as I stumbled into their fields during the 1980s. While I am now an Affiliate Professor of Psychiatry and Behavioral Sciences at the University of Washington, I am no more a psychiatrist now than I was a neurosurgeon before. Pressed for a specialization, I usually say that I'm a theoretical neurophysiologist trying to work out the neural circuitry for higher intellectual function – and that periodically leads me astray into linguistics and into the interrelationship between abrupt climate change and human origins.

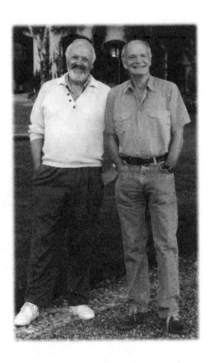

William H. Calvin   Derek Bickerton

DEREK BICKERTON

Although I graduated from the University of Cambridge, England in 1949, it wasn't until the 1960s that I entered academic life, first as a lecturer in English Literature at the University of Cape Coast, Ghana, and then, after a year's postgraduate work in linguistics at the University of Leeds, as Senior Lecturer in Linguistics at the University of Guyana (1967-71) – the "Senior" was perhaps due to my being the only linguist in the entire country! It was there that I developed a long-lasting interest in creole languages, and this, after a year at the University of Lancaster in England, brought me to Hawaii, where what is locally called "pidgin" is in fact a creole. For twenty-four years I was a Professor of Linguistics at the University of Hawaii, having meanwhile received a Ph.D. in linguistics from the University of Cambridge (1976). My work in Hawaii, and in particular my discovery that creole languages were produced by children from unstructured input in a single generation, led me to wonder where language had originally come from, and how it had developed to its present complexity. This led to an apprenticeship similar to Bill's – a learning experience that involved struggling with a variety of unfamiliar disciplines. But I'm a card-carrying autodidact, and I've always found boundaries oppressive, whether of countries, institutions, or academic disciplines. Crossing them has given me some of the most rewarding experiences of my life.

About the Artist

MARK MEYER, who did the cover art, is also a neurobiologist in the Department of Zoology at the University of Washington. Other examples of his art, and guides to his recent paintings, can be found at *http://3dotstudio.com*.

Terrence W. Deacon of Harvard Medical School and Boston University kindly photographed the bonobo and human brains that appear on the cover; we have kept their relative sizes unchanged. The Daniel C. Dennett quote is from *Kinds of Minds: Toward an Understanding of Consciousness* (Basic Books, 1996), p. 147.

WilliamCalvin@alum.mit.edu
http://faculty.washington.edu/wcalvin

Derek.Bickerton@worldnet.att.net

Supplements and corrections can be found on the web page
http://WilliamCalvin.com/LEM

Index

The **boldface** numerals indicate an entry in the glossary.